Retirement Abroad

Born in Cornwall in 1929, Robert Cooke has travelled and worked extensively in all five continents, visiting more than half the countries in the world. After twelve years in the Royal Navy his professional qualification in finance and administration led him into a business career with large groups of multinational companies. He worked in Saudi Arabia and for aid organizations in Uganda and the Sudan in the early 1980s and in 1987 he became a permanent resident on the Costa Blanca in Spain, where he is an independent financial consultant.

RETIREMENT ABROAD

*A Practical Guide to Retiring
in Another Country*

ROBERT COOKE, F.C.I.S.

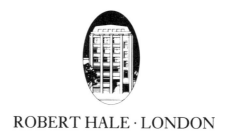

ROBERT HALE · LONDON

© *Robert Harlan Vivian Cooke 1993*
First published in Great Britain 1993

ISBN 0 7090 5026 7

Robert Hale Limited
Clerkenwell House
Clerkenwell Green
London EC1R 0HT

Photoset in Ehrhardt by
Derek Doyle & Associates, Mold, Clwyd.
Printed in Great Britain by
St Edmundsbury Press Ltd, Bury St Edmunds, Suffolk.
Bound by WBC Bookbinders Ltd, Bridgend, Mid-Glamorgan.

Contents

Acknowledgements

Many people of various nationalities have assisted in the research preparatory to writing this book, whether knowingly and consciously or unwittingly as a result of my observations of them. Whichever it is I thank them for their assistance.

In particular my special gratitude goes out to Emilio Salar Gálvez, Gestor Administrativo Colegiado, of Torrevieja, for checking the whole of the section on Spain and for providing up-to-date details of Spanish taxation. Michael Imison Playwrights Ltd very kindly gave permission for all the lyrics of Noël Coward's 'Mad Dogs and Englishmen' to be reprinted in Chapter 14. James Ivison read the manuscript and gave me the benefit of his experience in conducting pre-retirement courses. Canadians Iris and Joe Uriate did likewise to provide a North American perspective. P-E International plc of Park House, Wick Road, Egham, Surrey kindly supplied their latest index of living costs, details from which appear in Chapter 2.

1 Reasons for Retirement Overseas

Retirement is one of the three ages of man – and woman too for that matter. In our youth most of us are under the direction of our parents, who control our early life. Later the majority of us find that earning a living is a very demanding occupation; working and travelling into the evening; Saturdays busy with shopping and household chores; Sundays a day of rest and recuperation in preparation for the week ahead. This pattern is only broken by an occasional holiday, much of which is often taken up with unwinding from the stresses of modern living. It is only in retirement that most of us for the first time in our lives can do whatever we want to and go wherever we please. Of course, we can only do this if we have sufficient income and capital, making it mandatory to consider at an early age financial planning for retirement. Do not rely solely on a state pension to supply all your needs, as in most industrialized countries retired persons are representing an increasingly large proportion of the population and the economically active section is having to support a greater burden. The result is that state retirement pensions are unlikely to be generous and they may well be at or below the poverty level. There is nothing worse than having a lot of spare time on your hands and no available money to do anything interesting with it.

Why do people want to retire to a country which is different from that of their birth? One reason as stated above is that they are free to go wherever they want to within the limitations imposed by their wealth and the regulations of foreign governments. Another explanation may be that they want a complete change after the conclusion of their working lives, although this could be achieved by lengthy and frequent holidays. In fact, the possible reasons are probably as varied as the people retiring overseas, although a number of distinct and

11

recognizable patterns are evident in a large number of cases. Probably foremost amongst these are a search for a better climate, improved health, lower taxation, more economical living costs and a wider range of available activities; although this list is certainly far from exhaustive. Nevertheless, these are matters of such deep importance to almost all retired expatriates that they are worthy of special consideration.

Climate is discussed in more detail in the next chapter. Improved health may be physical or psychological. Make no mistake about it, stress is a serious killer. The cause of death on the certificate may read 'heart attack', but the question is what caused it? The answer is very often stress at work or in connection with domestic affairs. If stress is likely to continue after retirement then you are probably well advised to get right away from it into a fresh lifestyle. But be careful that you are not moving into a noisy environment or similar problems may recur. I have worked in London for various periods, but after a while I invariably said to myself, 'I have to get out of this madness, I can't stand it any longer'. Turning to the area where I live now, the World Health Organization has stated that the Costa Blanca region of Spain is one of the healthiest in the world. Here previous sufferers from arthritis and similar medical complaints adversely affected by cold and damp weather feel immediate benefit and many throw away walking sticks or even crutches. People from the northern countries which are mostly cloudy feel pleasure from lying in the sun, although it is the badly needed rest which is probably doing them the most good. If your one and only reason for retirement overseas is to sunbathe then consider your position very carefully, because after the first few weeks you would soon become bored with doing that all day and chronic melancholia could well result. It is vitally important to have sufficient activities to interest you. In any case, the depletion of the ozone layer has made sunbathing a hazardous lifestyle and if you indulge in it you should consider purchasing one of the new sunshades which have been developed to screen out ultraviolet light. In Australia one person in three is being treated for skin cancer, often necessitating operations.

Only a decade or two ago average life expectancy for a male person living in Britain was about 68 years, so retiring at 65 did not leave a very long period to be concerned about. Now with improved medicine, 'spare part' surgery developments and a healthier lifestyle as well as climate, many more people can expect to live well into their eighties. Although you may be alive at an advanced age you may not be particularly physically active and this is a future development to which you should give consideration in your advance planning. In many popular retirement countries a relative is expected to give support to a sick person and this can be a problem for a lone retiree. Even couples have to bear in mind that eventually one spouse will be alone. Sheltered homes are a possible solution and you should ensure that your finances will cover this alternative if it may become desirable.

I am not a doctor and if you are contemplating retirement abroad for health reasons then you should consult with your general practitioner concerning suitable locations. If you are in good health and considering a more exotic retirement base than Europe then you may find my experience of living and working in many parts of the world useful. All I can do in this part of the book is to give a general résumé on a continental basis. North America is mostly free from health hazards, although the cost of medical care in the USA and Canada is astronomical and generous insurance cover for treatment is a prerequisite. Mexico's main failing is lack of safe drinking water, but this should cause you only occasional and minor problems if care is exercised. In country areas medical facilities are extremely rudimentary, with often not even a stretcher available. Brazil is almost as big as the whole of Europe and has health standards as varied as its regions; generally lowest in the north (with yellow fever in southern Amazonia) and highest in the temperate south. Other parts of South America and Central America are reasonably healthy places to live, except for jungle areas, although the current cholera epidemic may well become widespread. Turning now to Africa, the north-west is moderately healthy with few problems. West Africa was long known as 'the white man's grave' and even though conditions have improved it still rates lowest, together with the whole Zaïre basin of the central area. The Horn of Africa also has a low rating, with the remainder of East Africa being rather better. The most healthy regions are Southern Africa and the Central Highlands. The desert areas, together with NE Africa, Arabia and the Near East should be avoided by those who may develop lung problems due to the continuous dust in the atmosphere.

The Middle East is unhealthy around the big river basins. Southern Asia varies with the arrival of the unpleasant monsoon season and the memsahibs of the Raj knew the value of altitude in the hill stations at such times. In SE Asia you just have to suffer the monsoon and its problems. Eastern Asia has a much healthier climate. There should be few difficulties in Australasia. Oceania is tropical and the health risks of the tropics should be expected.

Taxation is of such major interest to expatriates that it deserves a later chapter to itself. The subject of living costs is elaborated in Chapter 5. As regards activities, many possibilities are listed in Chapters 17, 18 and 19 and you should consider very carefully how you are going to spend your time in retirement. Oversimplifying as usual, I divide people into two categories – talkers and doers. If you are just a talker then it is essential to ensure that you will have similar company around you, otherwise you are very likely to earn a reputation as being 'that person who never has anything to do and wants to talk all day'. This would result in you soon wearing out your welcome. Property is certainly not cheap on the Costa del Sol of southern Spain, but developers have realized that retired people do not want just to sit around 'waiting to die' and they have provided a range of facilities on many urbanizations.

Who is unlikely to make a success of retirement abroad? The most severe problems are likely to be encountered by those who have lived almost all their lives in a small close community of mostly lifelong friends. Those with a highly developed sense of consumerism who want to spend much of the time shopping could experience difficulty if they choose a country with a less market-oriented economy than the one with which they are familiar. People who spend all their time denigrating their new country of abode and its institutions by continually making unfavourable comparisons with their own state will just make themselves unhappy. You have to accept your adopted country as it is, with all its imperfections, because you cannot change it. Possibly less serious, although leading to a lower level of enjoyment of retirement, are failure to study the new language, lack of interest in the new culture, alcoholism, financial problems caused by failure to plan a defence against inflation and depreciation of your home currency, noise and clashing lifestyles between residents and holidaymakers in mixed developments. Most of these more minor problems are avoidable with care and advance planning. Many people who are unhappy in a particular country or location may well have enjoyed their retirement in a different state or place. The purpose of this book is to bring out the good and bad points affecting retirement so that you become aware of them in advance and you can then avoid the pitfalls. Serious mistakes can often prove difficult or impossible to rectify and at worst can leave you with an unsaleable property which prevents you from moving elsewhere or even returning to your home country.

2 Selecting Possible Countries

As far as the range of countries available for retirement is concerned, the world is your oyster. The main limiting factors are insufficient finance and the immigration rules imposed by various states. Even the latter are often not taken too seriously by many retired people, because they ignore or circumvent the regulations. My advice is to respect immigration procedures for peace of mind and security of tenure of the property which you have purchased. It may seem difficult to believe, but wherever you go in the world you will find many retired people of different nationalities living there. Consequently it is sensible to give serious consideration to all the possibilities. If you asked me which country has all the advantages and no disadvantages as a retirement home then I should have to answer that I am still looking for it and I have not yet found it. If I do discover it I may not publicize the fact, as that could spoil it! The main problem I find is that there are seasonal variations and perhaps the solution is to regard your retirement home as a base which does not prevent you from spending part of each year in other countries if your finances permit.

Residence regulations vary for every country of the world and they are constantly changing, so I cannot give details in this book. The relevant embassy or consulate in your home country will supply full information. Not all countries expect immigrants to purchase property there and many are satisfied with a long-term tenancy agreement. Almost all states will not be too concerned with your amount of capital, but they will want proof that you are bringing into the country on a regular basis a minimum level of income which they regard as sufficient to support you. For instance, in Spain this figure is currently about 114,000 pesetas per month for a single person or 140,000 pesetas for a couple, although they normally accept anyone in receipt of a pension. In countries where as a permanent resident you are not entitled to free health care under reciprocal arrangements with your home country, because you are below the official minimum age for retirement for instance, then you are likely to be required to obtain health insurance cover. If you find that you cannot meet the requirements for permanent immigration then you may be satisfied with residence for six months in each year in those countries where your stay can legally be extended for this length of time. Those people from the European Community who believe that the other eleven states are an open house now may be in for a disappointment. Many of these countries are still operating the regulations very strictly and you should remember that EC rules only permit you to seek work in another member state or to retire in it after having worked in that country. There is no automatic right to permanent residence in another member state in other circumstances.

Your next question may well be, 'How much does it cost to purchase a property abroad?' Again I cannot give figures for every country of the world, although it may help to list below the minimum costs of property in the popular retirement areas. Obviously the upper limit is whatever you want to pay. However, if the minimum is above your means then that country can be eliminated from your consideration. Inflation will ensure that prices rise in local currency at least.

Sterling	Property	Local currency
ANDORRA		
£25,000	Studio apartment	*French Franc* 250,000
£38,000	Apartment, 1 bedroom	380,000
£47,000	Apartment, 2 bedrooms	470,000
£95,000	Town house, 3 bedrooms	950,000
£125,000	Chalet, 3 bedrooms	1,250,000
CYPRUS		
£20,000	Apartment, 1 bedroom	*Cyprus pound* 16,700
£25,000	Apartment or converted country house, 2 bedrooms	20,900
£30,000	Terraced bungalow, 2 bedrooms	25,000
£40,000	Detached villa, 2 bedrooms	33,400

Sterling	Property	Local currency

FRANCE
Brittany, Normany, Pas de Calais and Loire

£20,000	Town house, 2 bedrooms	*Franc* 200,000
£25,000	Cottage, 2 bedrooms	250,000
£50,000	Country house, 4 bedrooms	500,000

Charente

£15,000	Village house, 2 bedrooms	150,000
£40,000	Country house, 3 bedrooms	400,000

Charente Maritime

£25,000	Village house, 2 bedrooms	250,000
£50,000	Country house, 3 bedrooms	500,000

Dordogne and Lot

£30,000	Village house, 2 bedrooms	300,000
£35,000	Country cottage, 2 bedrooms	350,000
£40,000	Country house, 3 bedrooms	400,000
£50,000	Farm cottage, 3 bedrooms	500,000

Provence

£40,000	Village house, 2 bedrooms	400,000
£60,000	Country house, 3 bedrooms	600,000

Riviera

£35,000	Studio apartment	350,000
£70,000	Apartment, 1 bedroom	700,000
£100,000	Apartment, 2 bedrooms	1,000,000

GREECE
Mainland

£25,000	Apartment, 1 bedroom	*Drachma* 7,500,000
£30,000	Apartment, 2 bedrooms	9,000,000
£40,000	Villa, 2 bedrooms	12,000,000

Islands

£16,000	Studio apartment	4,800,000
£20,000	Apartment, 1 bedroom	6,000,000
£40,000	Villa, 2 bedrooms	12,000,000
£80,000	Town house, 2 bedrooms	24,000,000

IRELAND

£15,000	Country cottage (unmodernized), 2 bedrooms	*Punt* 16,500
£25,000	Country cottage (renovated), 2 bedrooms	27,500
£60,000	Country house, 4 bedrooms	65,800

Sterling	Property	Local currency

ITALY (All prices are for restored properties)
Umbria

£20,000	Apartment, 1 bedroom	*Lire* 44,000,000
£25,000	Cottage, 2 bedrooms	55,000,000
£35,000	Farmhouse, 3 bedrooms	77,000,000

Tuscany

£30,000	Village house, 1 bedroom, or	
	country cottage, 2 bedrooms	66,000,000
£75,000	Farmhouse, 2 bedrooms	165,000,000

MALTA
Main island

£25,000	Town apartment, 2 bedrooms	*Maltese pound* 14,550
£30,000	Converted village house,	
	17,450	3 bedrooms
£55,000	Semi-detached town house,	
	3 bedrooms	32,000
£75,000	Detached town house,	
	3 bedrooms	43,650

Gozo island

£20,000	Apartment, 2 bedrooms	11,650
£50,000	Semi-detached bungalow,	
	3 bedrooms	29,100
£55,000	Villa, 3 bedrooms	32,000

PORTUGAL

£25,000	Apartment, 1 bedroom	*Escudo* 6,450,000
£30,000	Apartment, 2 bedrooms	7,730,000
£55,000	Villa, 2 bedrooms	14,170,000

SPAIN
Cost Blanca

£16,000	Apartment, 1 bedroom	*Peseta* 2,900,000
£17,500	Apartment, 2 bedrooms	3,170,000
£18,000	Terraced bungalow, 1 bedroom	3,260,000
£20,000	Terraced bungalow, 2 bedrooms	3,620,000
£32,000	Villa, 2 bedrooms	5,790,000

Costa Brava

£30,000	Apartment, 1 bedroom	5,430,000
£35,000	Apartment, 2 bedrooms	6,340,000
£60,000	Villa, 2 bedrooms	10,860,000

Sterling	Property	Local currency
Costa de Almeria		
£15,000	Apartment, 1 bedroom	2,715,000
£30,000	Apartment, 2 bedrooms	5,430,000
£35,000	Terraced bungalow, 2 bedrooms	6,340,000
£65,000	Villa, 3 bedrooms	11,765,000
Costa del Sol		
£25,000	Apartment, 1 bedroom, or Village house, 2 bedrooms	4,525,000
£30,000	Country house, 2 bedrooms	5,430,000
£35,000	Apartment, 2 bedrooms	6,340,000
£120,000	Villa, 3 bedrooms	21,720,000
Majorca		
£15,000	Studio apartment	2,715,000
£20,000	Apartment, 1 bedroom	3,620,000
£25,000	Apartment, 2 bedrooms	4,525,000
£30,000	Bungalow, 2 bedrooms	5,430,000
£110,000	Country house, 3 bedrooms	19,910,000
Minorca		
£40,000	Apartment, 2 bedrooms	7,240,000
£50,000	Villa, 2 bedrooms	9,050,000
Ibiza		
£25,000	Apartment, 1 bedroom	4,525,000
£28,000	Apartment, 2 bedrooms	5,068,000
£75,000	Villa, 2 bedrooms	13,575,000
Canary Islands		
£25,000	Apartment, 1 bedroom, or small unconverted farmhouse with land	4,525,000
£32,000	Apartment, 2 bedrooms	5,790,000
£35,000	Bungalow, 2 bedrooms	6,340,000
£60,000	Villa, 2 bedrooms	10,860,000
TURKEY		
£12,000	Apartment, 1 bedroom	*Lira* 65,900,000
£14,000	Apartment, 2 bedrooms	76,885,000
£20,000	Villa, 3 bedrooms	109,835,000

The main variable in almost all cases is proximity to a beach. Dilapidated properties can often be purchased for approximately half of the above figures in a number of countries. This can be a good alternative if you have building experience or if you are a competent handyman. However, if you are going to pay for all the restoration work then it is doubtful whether you will make any saving. Do not necessarily assume that properties in countries which are more distant than those popular ones listed above are out of your reach as regards cost. For instance, if you favour retiring to the USA a very nice detached property on an ample plot can be purchased in Florida for about £28,000, although the problem is being allowed to live there for more than six months in a year.

Some people retire abroad mainly for reasons of taxation. This is perfectly understandable for natives of countries such as Sweden where the minimum level of taxation is likely to be about 50 per cent of income. Do not necessarily assume that taxes will be less in a foreign country than your own, because this may not be so when you check the system and figures. In fact, some may be higher and others lower, so consider which are more important to your circumstances; income tax, wealth tax, inheritance tax, value added tax, etc. Obtain as much detail as possible in advance concerning your intended country of residence. This information is always available from the relevant embassy or consulate, although you may need to be persistent to obtain full details. Then study the later chapter in this book headed 'Taxation' and do your calculations. This is important because of the way in which tax is levied. For example, both Britain and Spain had a minimum rate of income tax at 25 per cent, but Britain gives personal allowance against gross income whereas in Spain they are set against tax due, the latter being much more beneficial. Give careful consideration to where tax is going to be levied; it is pointless to select a nil tax state such as Andorra for retirement if your income will continue to arise in your home country and be fully taxed there. In fact, taxes may be levied upon you in two different countries and then it is important to ensure that a double taxation treaty is in existence between them, so that you can offset taxes paid in one state against taxes due in another.

Many countries also have reciprocal arrangements for paying state pensions to expatriates. For instance, Britain has concluded agreements with the following states:

Australia	Guernsey	Mauritius
Austria	Iceland	Netherlands
Belgium	Ireland	New Zealand
Bermuda	Italy	Norway
Canada	Isle of Man	Portugal
Cyprus	Israel	Spain
Denmark	Jamaica	Switzerland
Finland	Jersey	Turkey
France	Luxembourg	USA
Germany	Malta	Yugoslavia

It may be possible to make payments in other countries, so contact your social security office. A word of warning: if you retire in either Australia, Canada, New Zealand or Norway you will not receive the annual increase based on the UK rate of inflation, but your pension will remain fixed at the figure originally granted. As the recent rate of annual inflation was 8.6 per cent in Australia and 5 per cent in Canada, you will see that the value of your pension will rapidly depreciate.

Which naturally leads us on to the subject of inflation, again of enough importance to deserve a later chapter. Staying with state pensions for the moment, it is vital to appreciate that even if you do receive an annual increase, this will be based upon the inflation rate in your country of origin and not the country of residence. Therefore if the inflation rate is higher in the latter than the former then you will need to fund the difference by such means as investments, in order to preserve your standard of living.

This seems to be flowing quite well because we next have to consider the cost of living in the country of intended residence. This can vary enormously and costs can easily be three times as high in one country as another. For example, the following is a comparison of average expatriate living costs (excluding housing on the assumption that a retired person will be buying and not renting property) at October 1991, taking Britain as the base of 100:

Japan	145	Greece	93
Norway	129	Australia	91
Sweden	124	Canada	91
Finland	121	Grenada	91

Switzerland	112	Luxembourg	89
Denmark	111	Netherlands	89
Italy	104	Portugal	88
Bahamas	102	Malta	87
France	102	USA	86
Belgium	101	Cyprus	85
Hong Kong	101	Trinidad	85
Seychelles	101	New Zealand	78
Spain	101	Fiji	75
Austria	100	Mexico	73
UK	100	Morocco	71
Ireland	97	Cost Rica	61
Germany	94	India	54
Barbados	93	Jamaica	44

Do not necessarily take too much notice of figures issued by the countries themselves because they are usually based upon costs for their own nationals who frequently have a different spending pattern from expatriates, besides paying lower prices for the same thing! Unless you have relations or friends resident in the country who can give you reliable information, then there is no real substitute for renting property there (see Chapter 5) and discovering costs for yourself.

I cannot stress too strongly that ignoring the effects of inflation in your country of retirement can easily be a matter of life and death. At worst it could mean that you do not have enough money for sufficient food on which to live. Therefore you should give very careful consideration to this vital subject which is discussed fully in chapter 27, making plans for dealing with this matter before it becomes serious.

Climate is always an important factor in selecting a place for retirement, whether it is for psychological reasons or for practical ones such as lower fuel costs. Be certain to do your research carefully by visiting the intended country of residence at three different times of the year. You would probably be amazed that a high proportion of the people who emigrate to Spain do not even realize that this country can be cold in winter. This is because all their previous visits on vacations have been during the summer season. Life can be very different in a country when the climate changes from that found during July and August. Most places take on a very different character for the remainder of the year and at worst they can be ghost towns for ten months. Remember that there is nowhere in mainland Europe where you can guarantee warm weather in winter. However, careful attention to situation and aspect in selecting a property for purchase (as discussed in Chapter 6) can make permanent life very pleasant in many Mediterranean regions. If you are looking for the certainty of a warm winter climate then you need to go as far south as the Canary Islands. Remember that in the southern hemisphere, south of the equator, the seasons are reversed and summer is centred around January in countries such as Brazil and Australia.

The social aspects of language should not be underestimated in deciding upon a country for retirement. Many elderly people say that it is too late in life for them to learn a new language, or that their memory is now very poor. The importance of exercising your brain and your memory cannot be overstressed. If you are prepared to make some attempt at learning the local language then you are not likely to experience problems of this kind. If not, then you could become very lonely and depressed about not being able to carry on a conversation. This is likely to be a greater difficulty in country areas, which are not so cosmopolitan as the coast. Some people solve this problem by emigrating to a country which speaks their language, such as the British retiring to Malta or the Portuguese to Brazil. The alternative is to select an expatriate community which contains a number of people of your own nationality.

Finally, the closeness of your home ties may well influence your choice of retirement location. If you have parents, children or grandchildren remaining in your country of origin then the ease, frequency and cost of transport to visit them will be an important consideration. In such a situation you may well opt for a country where cheap return flights are available for around £60, rather than retire to Mauritius where the cost is likely to be about £1,000 per trip to Europe. Although some working adults or their spouses are prepared to take responsibility for looking after aged parents, many find this an intolerable burden and you should aim to be self-reliant in retirement.

3   Information Gathering

Long before you get down to the task of deciding upon a retirement location you should make a start on gathering details of possible countries. A great deal of information is available and much of it is completely free. A vast amount of data is available in embassies and consulates, although generally they cannot be bothered with you and will attempt to brush you off with the absolute minimum, particularly if your enquiry is by telephone or letter. If possible make a personal call, be charming to the official about his or her country and certainly do not adopt an aggressive attitude, demanding information as of right.

Tourist offices in your home country are considerably more helpful in most cases. In order to assist them to help you it is essential to supply full details of your range of interest, particularly for telephonic and postal enquiries. Better still, go to the office and help yourself to the literature displayed there. The standard can be very variable, from translations into your language which are barely understandable to superbly illustrated leaflets which contain an enormous amount of useful information. Nevertheless, you should be aware that their function is to sell holidays in that country and it is looked at through rose-coloured spectacles to varying extents from a slight manipulation of the facts to downright lies. Anyway, it is all free, so what have you to lose? If writing to a tourist office outside your home country it is advisable to enclose sufficient International Reply Coupons, obtainable from your post office.

There are many excellent single country guides available from bookshops and many others which are not very good. If it is obvious from the jacket that the author is a journalist resident in your own country then they could have picked up a smattering of information on a few brief visits which may or may not be accurate, making the book of doubtful use. On the other hand if the author is a professional person resident in the country in question then the chances are of a much higher standard of information. If you are contemplating retirement in Spain you may care to consider my first book entitled *A Villa on the Costa Blanca*, which is obtainable by sending a cheque for £9 payable to Mrs N. Taylor at 13 Dee Avenue, Kilmarnock, Scotland.

You should not confine your research just to guides. If the country is to be your new home it is also important to have an understanding of its culture, history and politics, not to mention such subjects as its art and traditional cooking. Reference libraries contain a wealth of information on such topics and the index is likely to be on a geographical basis making selection a simple matter. Lending libraries, depending upon size, may well contain a very restricted choice in comparison, particularly as many of the books likely to be of interest to you are published only in paperback format which they do not stock. Nevertheless, there are probably non-fiction books available in your library which will supply background information.

Although it is sensible to collect as many details as possible in your home country there is no real substitute for visiting the place you have in mind for retirement. Apart from being an opportunity to obtain on the spot information it will also enable you to form impressions of the country and to decide whether it 'feels right', which is very important. There are three main ways in which you can achieve this. You may make a journey for this specific reason; perhaps take a vacation and combine the two; or there could be the possibility of an inspection flight organized by a property promoter. You may take the first alternative because there is some urgency, such as the fact that you have just sold your house at home and have nowhere to live. Personally I advise strongly against rushing into a selection in this hurried fashion and suggest that you should go through the sequence of vacations and renting property in the target country. Nevertheless, it sometimes happens that it is necessary to decide quickly, such as times when property is escalating rapidly in price and it could soon be outside your budget. In such circumstances it is essential to go armed with a preparatory list of information which you will need. Property prices and purchasing costs, details of estate agencies, the name, address and telephone number of a local solicitor having a staff who speak your language, your local consulate, costs of electricity, gas and water, and how to open an account with a local bank are just a few of the details which you are certain to require. If combined with a vacation, then this information can be obtained in a more leisurely fashion; although you should be well aware of the temptation to spend the days sleeping on the beach with the result that you may leave all the work until the last day only to find it is a public holiday and everywhere is closed. It is much better to work through a proportion of your list each day commencing with the priority items. An inspection flight may well suit your purpose, particularly if preliminary indications are that you are very likely to purchase from one specific building promoter. Generally no pressure is exerted to buy, they are well organized and the cost may be subsidised. However, you should be aware that it is the purchaser who eventually provides the subsidy and the person who does not buy is the one who receives the benefit. If you consider that an inspection flight will be an opportunity to investigate all the possibilities then you are wasting your time as the promoter has a vested interest in ensuring that you have no opportunity to see anything other than what he has to offer.

4 Preparatory Holidays

Bearing in mind my earlier warning that seasonal changes in many resorts can be considerable, vacations in the country you have in mind for retirement can still be a very useful preparation. Even so, you need to transpose your mind from tourist to resident and see matters through different eyes. Some things may be bearable for a few weeks, but how will they seem when you have to endure them on a permanent basis? The following are just some of the subjects that you may want to consider as a resident while you are experiencing the quite different life of a tourist.

During your vacation you may well be hiring a car and this is something that you are not likely to do as a resident for very long, if for no other reason than that it would be too expensive. If you are likely to buy a car later then it would be useful to compare prices and see what guarantees are given in order to obtain a feel for the local market. If you are not going to drive then it is important to know exactly what public transport services exist. Train services are unlikely to fulfil all your needs, whether they are good, infrequent or non-existent. So you need to study the bus schedules, costs, frequency, adequacy and comfort of services, as well as whether they only operate on a seasonal basis. Taxi rates may be relevant in some situations. You should remember that in a hot climate it may be quite exhausting for an elderly person to walk comparatively short distances which cause no problem at home in cooler weather. Those who intend to drive at first should bear in mind that later on advancing years may result in them being unable to retain a licence and continue to drive.

If you are spending your vacation in a hotel all your meals may be provided and consequently your main shopping requirements could be confined to buying some souvenirs to take home. Even so, it can be very informative to walk through the larger shops and supermarkets, even if you purchase little or nothing. The same is true of open air markets, where fruit and vegetables are usually a bargain, even if other things are a tourist 'rip off'. It is not difficult to imagine your weekly menus and then see how much the ingredients would cost so that you have an approximate weekly budget. Of course, this does not tell you how rapidly prices are rising, but if you make more than one visit and take notice of the costs at different times then you will have an idea of the true inflation rate.

In the situation of full board at a hotel there will probably be no need for you to have a meal at a restaurant. Nevertheless, it is a simple matter to look at the boards displayed at the entrance, besides taking note of what savings can be made by opting for the meal of the day which often includes wine. However, do not make the mistake of a friend of mine in Cannes who remarked after studying the menu of a restaurant on the seafront, 'Even the poison is expensive here!' He was looked at *poisson* (fish).

Local sports facilities may well be used by visitors and quite possibly they could be of the type which are likely to appeal to residents. This is an area where the tourist office in the town can provide a great deal of information and no doubt they will have maps available so that you can go and check out the possibilities. You will also need to consider costs, as the occasional spending of a visitor may not be possible on a regular basis for retired people on a budget. Certain sports such as golf are often quite expensive to follow because it is costly to use large quantities of water to maintain the greens and fairways in a good condition in a dry climate.

Local entertainments are equally likely to appeal both to visitors and expatriates. These can only be provided on a commercial basis at times when there are sufficient customers to make them economic, so enquire from local people you meet what entertainment is likely to be available outside the normal tourist season. Discovering the range of entertainments should not be too difficult as, besides the tourist office, you probably will find free newspapers or leaflets, as well as information in your hotel lobby. Remember too that there are likely to be many free entertainments throughout the year, such as folklore festivals and fiestas. They are usually well worth seeing and it pays to search for a calendar of local events; even though you may not want to run through the streets of Pamplona ahead of the bulls!

Television is a cheap form of entertainment which many people spend a considerable time watching in their home country; perhaps far more than they realize. In a hotel you are able to see the local programmes, although they are likely to be of little interest if you do not speak the language, except possibly for some musical and sports items. I do not think a person should allow television to rule his or her life, but if it is very important to you as a form of entertainment and likely to affect the enjoyment of your retirement, then it could have considerable bearing upon where you decide to purchase a property. In an isolated or detached situation the only means of obtaining additional programmes is very likely to be by purchasing a satellite receiving dish costing £1,000 or more. If this is beyond your budget it may be desirable to consider buying a property on an urbanization, where cable television is part of the infrastructure and there is a much smaller connection fee, or perhaps only a monthly maintenance charge. For instance, I have a choice of twenty channels in Spain, including four in German, five in Spanish, two in French, two in Swedish and six in English. Five of the latter are produced by British Sky Broadcasting and the remaining BBC World Service station has mainly BBC1 programmes plus a few from BBC2.

5 Renting Property

A much better insight into expatriate lifestyle can be obtained by renting property in the target country rather than staying in a hotel. This way, there may be no difference whatsoever except for the proviso that the stay is temporary as opposed to permanent. Of course, it may not be possible in some locations to rent exactly where you wish to buy for reasons such as rents may be within your budget but property is too expensive for you to purchase, or that properties are available for sale but not for rental. Also you may well feel that you have different needs for holidays and permanent residence and renting in an area suitable for the latter may detract from your enjoyment of your vacation.

Property built specifically for holidaymakers may well be quite unsuitable for permanent residence. On vacation you tend to spend a great deal of time on the beach or sightseeing as well as at places of evening entertainment. In such circumstances an apartment to provide somewhere to sleep may be the main requirement. A permanent resident on the other hand is likely to spend a great deal more time at home and consequently have substantial interest that the accommodation provides adequate living space. Of particular concern will be comfort during the winter months, when the weather may well be cold.

You will also need to consider what facilities which are not provided or available in holiday accommodation are desirable or essential for permanent residence. You may feel that you need a telephone in order to keep in touch with relatives and friends in your country of origin. In this case choose the property which you are buying with care, as there can be a delay of many years in a number of locations for installation of a telephone. With advancing age you may want the proximity of a clinic to provide medical assistance. Postal services may not seem very important on vacation, but you may be concerned about the possibility of having to collect your mail for years before a delivery is commenced in the area.

The above are just a few of many possible examples of how different life is for the holidaymaker and the expatriate resident. In order to consider the differences in lifestyle you will need to shift your mind on to a different plane and try to imagine living there on a permanent basis. If you find that you can imagine day to day life in the country then this will give you an ideal opportunity to experience a brief foretaste of permanent residence.

Renting property also gives you an unsurpassed insight into living costs for the expatriate, because your shopping lists and checkout slips will provide incontrovertible evidence of expenditure on food and household items. The total may be slightly on the higher side, as you will gradually learn with experience to shop around for the best deals, whereas you may not bother to do this if you wish to rush off to the beach. In fact, identical articles may be sold at three different prices to nationals, expatriates and visitors. For instance, very few people know that in Spanish open air markets (other than for fruit and vegetables), price tickets often have a higher figure facing outwards and a lower price marked on the back for Spaniards. Of course, this short experience will not give you a good guide to the longer term expenses such as the costs of heating, cooking and lighting, besides rates and motoring expenditure.

6   Purchasing Property

An indication of minimum prices at the present time was given in Chapter 2 for property in various popular retirement areas. You should appreciate that there can be substantial variation in the cost of almost identical properties depending upon whether you deal with an agent in your home country or go to see the situation for yourself on the spot. The differential can be as high as 30 per cent in countries such as Italy. Of course, it is easy and comfortable to purchase through an agent at home, but this is 'lazy man's buying' and a method which you could well regret for a long time into the future. If you intend to emigrate to a foreign country then the sooner you become familiar with its institutions and procedures the better. Naturally, the latter approach does leave you more open to the risk of fraud, although this should be minimal if you follow the later imprecation in this chapter to take proper legal advice.

By this stage of the book you may have a few ideas on points to watch out for in purchasing a retirement home and likely countries for emigration. In selecting a property to buy I cannot stress too strongly that the three most important considerations are location, location and location. It is quite useless to find your ideal house if it is in the wrong place for the everyday needs of your lifestyle. So do make a list of the facilities which you consider to be either essential or desirable for the enjoyment of your retirement and consider carefully how the property is located in relation to those needs.

Because location is of such paramount importance we need to take it a step further and also consider situation within a particular location, which includes aspect. This does not only cover an evaluation of whether you are likely to enjoy an uninterrupted view of a brick wall or a seascape to rolling countryside. You should also give thought to whether you want resident neighbours for company, or the peace of surrounding properties which are seldom used. Noise, particularly at night, can be a very disturbing element in the life of retired people, whether it comes from traffic, nearby bars, holidaymakers or screaming children in a swimming pool. Aspect, too, is a very important consideration for your comfort and budget. Unless you go to a tropical country it is very likely to be cold in winter and you will want to obtain full benefit from the ample sunshine which is likely to be available. For instance, in Spain I deliberately chose a villa facing south-east as the morning winter sunshine comes into the living-room and I have warmth on the front veranda for most of the day; whereas the kitchen, which I want to be cooler, is on the north side. If your property faces west or north you could experience little or no effect from the sun and the result for most pensioners who lead inactive lives is very likely to be an expensive bill for heating costs in winter.

Never – but never – buy property abroad without first taking proper legal advice, firstly ensuring that the lawyer or notary is not also acting for the seller. Do not sign any document or make any payment, even of a deposit, until you have received the benefit of this advice. Without this guidance you do not know the legal effect of signing, as the document is very likely to be in a foreign language; even if it is not you are probably unfamiliar with the laws of the country in question. Similarly with payments, you may be used to property purchases being 'subject to contract' or for deposits to be returnable in certain circumstances, but very likely the laws of another state will be quite different. The two most important matters which you will want your lawyer or notary to confirm are that the contract is fair to you as the purchaser and that you are conveyed a clear and unencumbered title to the property. If the country has exchange control regulations, such as Portugal then your legal representative will explain the proper procedure for importation of funds. This is essential in case you may later want to sell the property and repatriate the funds. Failure to comply with the rules could very likely leave your proceeds frozen in the foreign country, or subject to a long delay of years before release. There is probably little point in asking your solicitor at home to handle the purchase, as that person would almost certainly appoint a local lawyer and so this just adds to costs. Your nearest consulate in the country of purchase should be able to recommend local lawyers who speak your language or have linguists on their staff. It is often normal to give such lawyers power of attorney to complete the acquisition if you are likely to be absent. However, you should ensure that the property will be registered in your name and not that of the lawyer or other person. This is because the laws of many countries do not recognize nominees and regard the registered person as the full beneficial owner.

The contract for the purchase of a property is a very important document and you should ask for a translation into a language which you understand, so that you can give very careful consideration to whether it meets with your complete and unqualified approval. Not only check the clauses which it contains but also be very aware of necessary safeguards which it omits. If the property is yet to be built then it is very important to include an onerous penalty clause for late completion by the promoter or builder. This is essential because time has no meaning in many countries and builders often start a great many projects to boost their cash flow, although they later make very little progress upon them. Substantial delay could well involve you in serious unexpected expense.

When considering your budget for the purchase of a property abroad you should appreciate that various charges are very likely to add a considerable sum to the purchase price. These could well amount to about 10 to 12 per cent of the cost, although there are wide variations in different circumstances and states, so fuller details for the popular retirement countries are given later. Charges cover such matters as value added tax or other fiscal impositions, registration fees, cost of deeds, notorial fees, as well as connection charges for electricity and water.

Which brings us to the question of how you pay for the property and the related expenses. If you are able to settle in cash then that is fine. Even if you are in that fortunate position you should still consider whether it would be to your advantage to take out a mortgage in order to reduce your tax liability. For instance, in Spain an expatriate resident under certain conditions can deduct mortgage interest each year against income tax due, which is much more advantageous than against gross income. However, professional advice should be taken to ensure that you comply with such rules as the funds must emanate from a locally registered company. If you need a mortgage in order to purchase a property abroad then funds may be available in your home country or in the foreign state in question. For example, a few British building societies make advances for property purchases on the Costa del Sol and they are planning to extend the facility to the Costa Blanca. Advances are not necessarily secured upon a property in your home country and it is frequently possible to obtain a mortgage secured on a foreign property. In the latter case maximum advances are typically in the region of 60 to 70 per cent of the valuation, although you may be fortunate enough to be advanced as much as 90 per cent. In many countries there is no real equivalent to the building society and most mortgage facilities in Continental Europe are provided by the commercial banks. Of course, in general retired people do not take on large liabilities of this sort late in their lives. These notes are mainly intended for younger people who are planning for their retirement by purchasing an overseas property before costs escalate beyond their means.

Foreign currency mortgages are frequently available to expatriates when they do not wish to borrow in their home currency and these may well be expressed in the currency of the country in which the property is situated, or there could be a choice of third currencies. So a Swedish person could buy a property in Portugal with a mortgage denominated in Swiss francs, to give just one possible example of many permutations. At this stage I must give a warning in the strongest possible terms that taking a foreign currency mortgage could have serious consequences for you, resulting not only in the loss of your overseas property, but necessitating the sale of your house at home as well to meet your liabilities. If sterling interest rates are very high it may seem like a good idea to take a mortgage in Swiss francs when the rate is 6 per cent less. Most people have no idea of the extent of the currency risk to which they are exposing themselves in these circumstances. Generally interest rates are high in countries with a weak currency and low in those with a strong currency. For instance, the Swiss franc has appreciated against sterling by 23 per cent over the past nine years. Movements can be much more rapid than that and the Spanish peseta has appreciated by over 16 per cent against sterling during the calendar year 1989. Professional advice should always be sought before accepting a foreign currency mortgage. Even then you should be aware that you are taking on a liability the possible extent of which cannot be estimated, because exchange rate fluctuations are often completely unpredictable. Even experts would probably be reasonably satisfied if their projections were correct 60 per cent of the time. The possible exposure is more serious when all of your income and capital is in one currency and the mortgage repayments in another. Of course, your risk is reduced if you have investments denominated in the same currency as the mortgage. Exchange rates are an important matter for expatriates and the subject deserves the separate chapter which follows later.

7 Furnishings

A high proportion of resale properties abroad are sold with furniture, as the seller does not want the considerable expense of moving it. The market price of second-hand furniture is likely to be very low if an attempt was made to sell it separately. For the purchaser this means that all the essentials of living are readily available at the outset. Undoubtedly the new owners will want to make changes because the furniture does not suit their tastes. In this situation my advice would be not to rush into immediate alterations and make expensive mistakes, but to be patient a little while longer and gain some experience of living in the country, so as to make the ideal purchases.

For those persons buying a new property from a developer it is very likely that a complete furniture package will be offered. The good features of a package deal are that it often represents excellent value because the developer is purchasing at wholesale prices and making a single large sale; also a number of free items are usually given as an inducement, which would cost a considerable amount if purchased separately. Another consideration for new owners anxious to move in as quickly as possible to avoid hotel charges or expensive rented accommodation is that a complete installation service is often provided free of charge. This can save a great deal of time as you may otherwise have to search in a strange country for tradesmen to do such jobs as hanging curtains, fixing light fittings and drilling holes for wall furnishings. The drawbacks to acceptance are that the purchasers cannot project their tastes and personalities upon the property, besides the fact that it may seem like a very regimented housing scheme where all the properties are identical and furnished alike. A compromise may be possible because promoters are often prepared to show a measure of flexibility regarding the contents of the standard package. For instance, a different three-piece suite can completely transform a 'package look' and the exclusion of the standard suite can possibly be compensated by other useful items of furniture. Whether or not you accept the deal it still pays to study the package list as the developer knows the exact requirements of the properties and this may highlight omissions of essentials on your own list as well as point out useless and unnecessary items.

How much will it cost to furnish a foreign property? This is a question impossible to answer with exactitude as a great deal depends upon quality, your taste, your budget and the country in which you are buying. To give one typical example, furniture is not expensive in Spain and you should be able to furnish a property adequately for comfort for around 12 per cent of the purchase price. Wherever you are buying always enquire before placing an order whether any discounts are available. There is often considerable competition between retailers in this market and they may well make a fair deduction to secure what is a high value sale subject to a wide trade margin. However, make certain of the normal price first to ensure that you really are being given a discount and that the figure is not being uplifted before being reduced by a sham discount to the normal price. Have a look at the stock of furniture warehouses where they sell directly to the public as their prices are frequently very competitive because they save on expensive showroom costs. Often they can supply variations in styles and patterns to order at fairly short notice.

Quite apart from any savings in cost, it is almost invariably better to buy your furniture locally because it is much more likely to be suited to the climate and lifestyle. Even so, it is important to check items such as chairs and beds for comfort, as the latter are frequently fitted with wooden slats rather than springs. Good quality slats may be recommended for medical reasons. When buying items such as washing machines and refrigerators in countries where quality control inspection is not of a high standard it is advisable to select brands with an international reputation. If you obtain these from a large department store the protection is likely to be greater. Remember when purchasing a refrigerator that in a hot climate you are likely to require a greater capacity than is normal in a cooler country. Before buying a freezer it is desirable to gain experience of the continuity of electricity supplies, as frequent power cuts can make this item useless. Another point which many people moving to a warmer climate do not appreciate is just how much time they are likely to spend on their terrace or verandah. Therefore it is important to consider adequate and comfortable furniture for this part of the property. Indoors, the problem of a hot or humid climate is likely to be perspiration stains and you should select patterns accordingly, besides considering the options for cleaning and washing. In sandy or dusty areas such as Southern Europe and North Africa remember that dark wood shows every speck of dust and so it is advisable to select light woodwork. In the former area although houses are built for coolness, with tiled floors and an air space below, you should have floor covering of adequate thickness to provide insulation in winter. Slippers with a thick sole can be of assistance in this respect, particularly in kitchen areas which you may not want to cover.

Unless you have your own van it is seldom worthwhile importing furniture from another country as, quite apart from the high cost of removal and any customs duties which may be imposed, it is quite likely that the furniture will not be suited to the new home. The best solution therefore is to attempt to sell your old house with furniture, or to send the latter to the sale-room for what it will fetch. Alternatively, copy the American idea and have a furniture sale in your garage. In the case of antiques it is advisable to take professional advice on whether the furniture is likely to become ruined or valueless in excessively dry or humid climates, besides the risks in tropical countries from termites and other pests. Even if you do dispose of all your furniture there are very likely to be personal effects which you are unable to transport with you. Advice on removal facilities abroad is given in Chapter 12.

8   Preparation for Retirement

The worst possible thing you can do is to work extremely hard right up to the day of your retirement and then suddenly find that you have nothing to do all day. This is a considerable shock to the mental and physical systems, which in severe cases could result in medical problems. Taking the mental adjustment first of all: if your lifestyle is going to change considerably in a new country, it is advisable very gradually to withdraw from the pubs and clubs which you may frequent and step by step take up the new sports and pastimes which you will follow in the future. Drawing an analogy with jet lag, I always mitigate its effects by resetting my watch to the time of the new country on boarding the aircraft, rather than just before leaving it. Do not underestimate the physical shock to your body on the change from work to retirement. If your job requires a fair amount of effort it is important not to stop the exercise suddenly or the limbs will tighten up and you may well become musclebound. Even in a sedentary job you may be surprised to learn just how much effort goes into travelling to and from work. The ideal approach is to have at least as much exercise initially in retirement as before and little by little reduce it to the level appropriate to your new lifestyle. I am not suggesting that you take up weight-lifting or even engage in jogging (which can be harmful in hot weather) but, depending upon the climate, you are likely to have healthy alternatives such as swimming, walking or cycling, the latter being very good for the circulation and the heart as long as you do not have to contend with steep hills or the dangers of traffic on narrow roads.

Another adjustment which you are likely to need to make is to your diet. In the case of moderately active persons a man needs about 3,000 calories per day and a woman 2,200. For sedentary people these figures are reduced to 2,500 and 2,000

respectively. In other words, a man in retirement who is not
active needs about 17 per cent less food and a woman 9 per cent
less than when working. What happens if you ignore this
reduced requirement for the body? The result is likely to be that
you will put on excess and unwanted fat which will be
self-multiplying, with the consequent harmful effects of strain
upon the heart and other medical problems. Sufficient books
have been written on diets to fill a whole library. My suggestion
is the very simple and effective one of reducing the staples;
bread and potatoes. In fact, during time working in Saudi Arabia
with lavish food and little opportunity for exercise in the
sweltering heat I cut bread and potatoes out of my diet
completely for a year. Most people retiring to a warmer climate
should find that this dietary adjustment is easily made by having
a salad lunch in place of a cooked meal. Keep a note of your
weight and check it at intervals to ensure that a gradual and
steady increase is not escaping your attention.

Planning the new lifestyle is something which you should do
consciously and not just drift into it, with the possible result in
the latter case of being sidetracked into a different pattern from
what you really desire. In the case of a couple, the planning
should be done together. During working life you may be
surprised at just how little time husband and wife spend
together. In retirement abroad this is very likely to change
considerably. It must be recognized that tensions may well arise
as a result and they are much less likely to be serious if they are
faced frankly from the start. To give just one example, the wife
may be in the habit of having 'coffee mornings' with women
friends, which the husband probably has never experienced and
of which he may be almost unaware. If such a gathering takes
place when the husband had planned to do something particular
in the house he may alienate the visitors through annoyance and
lack of hospitality, causing later recriminations from his wife for
the loss of her friends. Knowing in advance when the coffee
morning is going to take place and arranging to be out of the
house at that time could avoid this kind of problem. Husband
and wife may well want to spend time doing different things. It is
essential in retirement to have enough to do and sufficient to
interest you so that there is a good reason to get up in the
morning and to avoid drifting into a lethargic frame of mind.
Which brings us to the point that it is just as important to

stimulate the brain in retirement as the body, because the former controls the latter. The greatest mistake which you can make is to 'live in the past', as a senile mind is likely to follow. Enjoy the present and look to the future because you could very well have another twenty years ahead of you; so keep active in body and in mind.

Quite a number of popular sports and pastimes are listed in Chapter 18 as possible suggestions to occupy your time, although this list is far from exhaustive. If you are considering taking up a new hobby in retirement it is often a good idea to attempt it first in your own country. This way you will find clubs to advise and assist you, as well as the availability of books on the subject in your own language. Perhaps you are quite familiar with the pastime but it requires the participation of others to make it possible or enjoyable. In that case you should be quite prepared to form a club yourself if none exists already. All kinds of activities can be interesting and fun whether or not you have previous experience of them, be it baseball, stamp collecting, mountain walking or whatever.

9   Learning the Language

I cannot stress too strongly the danger of moving to a foreign country where you are unable to carry on a conversation with anyone except the person with whom you live, if any. This situation could very easily lead to acute depression and severe melancholia. Television or radio in your own language helps a little, although these forms of communication are no substitute for the exchange of words. So if you are not going to make any attempt to learn the local language perhaps the British are best advised to go to Malta or Cyprus, the Portuguese to Brazil and the French to Tahiti! Seriously though, language is a problem for elderly people, particularly for those who have difficulty in memorizing and its importance to the enjoyment of your retirement should not be underestimated. The impasse is solved by many people through going to live in a cosmopolitan area such as the Mediterranean resorts, or on a development where there are a number of people of their own nationality. Nevertheless some attempt should be made to learn the language, as you will find that local people appreciate your efforts even if they correct your mistakes. Keeping your mind and your memory active may well prolong your life.

Once you have decided upon retirement in a certain country it is never too early to commence learning the language, because if the time which you have available for this purpose is limited then it could take years to attain reasonable fluency. The first important point is to ensure that you are studying the correct language for your retirement area, as there may be more than one primary or secondary tongue spoken within a single country. For instance, if you are going to the Costa Brava or the Balearic Islands then Catalan, which is a separate language and not a dialect of Spanish, is used by the local people. In the Rif area of northern Morocco the secondary tongue is Spanish, although it is French for the remainder of the country. The main reason why an early commencement to your studies is desirable is the fact that facilities for learning the foreign language in your home country could well be better than possibilities which you may find after arrival abroad, strange as that may seem. Before moving abroad you may well find facilities for learning the required language at local evening classes. Some polytechnics organize intensive courses at various levels during vacation times. In addition you have commercial language schools in various locations, which are mostly very well administered. Your local reference library should be able to inform you regarding all the possibilities. In North America the Boards of Education organize classes in a wide range of languages.

Regarding the methods of teaching, most people will probably opt for evening classes, as the cost is low through subsidization by the local authority. It is important to join the course from the beginning when it commences in the autumn and where demand is great it is essential to enrol as soon as lists are open to ensure a place. Your progress is likely to be in inverse ratio to the number of students, as a teacher cannot give individual attention to the problems of a large number. A fair number of students are likely to drop out as the course progresses; but unfortunately, most authorities have rules which suspend classes when numbers fall below a certain level as they are no longer economic. A lot will depend also on the mix of experience which the students possess. Where a course is stated to be of elementary level and most of the students have some knowledge of the language then an absolute beginner may soon lose touch. Conversely, many students find progress frustratingly slow due to it being geared to the aptitude of the worst members of the class; so that some of the better ones look for a quicker alternative.

Of course, self-instruction can save you time and money in not having to travel to classes, as well as giving you the flexibility of studying whenever you wish. The latter advantage brings out the need for self-discipline to keep up a set level or progress. Make no mistake about it, learning a language is hard work and it is so much easier to say, 'I'd rather watch something on television this evening'. The serious danger in teaching yourself is the mispronunciation of words, a fault which is extremely difficult to correct later and can make your speech completely unintelligible to a foreigner. For this reason, if you are studying from a book it is essential to select one which gives a phonetic pronunciation for every word and even this is of limited assistance. Every opportunity should be taken to listen to radio broadcasts or television if you have satellite or cable services. This is important not only for reasons of pronunciation, but also to acquire the correct stress on the syllables as well as the rhythm of sentences, which is often overlooked even by commercial schools, although essential for correct understanding. For instance, English sentences rise gradually in rhythm to a level plateau and then drop at the end, unless a question is being asked when it rises. Spanish has a rat-tat-tat, rat-tat-tat, rat-tat-tat rhythm. In Arabic there are frequent jumpy variations from low to high points. My experience of teaching languages has shown me that the audio-visual method is incontestably by far the best. If you have a book and a tape you are learning not only by ears but also by eyes and the latter are far more efficient. A teacher at an evening class would probably be reasonably pleased if students retained about half of the vocabulary by the next lesson, whereas I have found consistently that students of the audio-visual method frequently retain 97 per cent of the vocabulary for three months or longer. And retention is what language teaching is all about, because it is no good learning words one day and forgetting them the next. You may be fortunate in finding a book and cassette set available on loan from your local public library.

Commercial language schools are mostly not subject to state inspection or control and as a result their efficiency tends to be very variable. If possible ensure that your teacher is a native speaker of the language which you wish to learn, as others can give only an approximate rendition of the pronunciation. Should you have a choice of schools then ask them about rhythm of the language and avoid those evasive or mystified by your questions. As an alternative to a school you may be able to arrange for private tuition, particularly in a city where there are likely to be teachers and students from other countries studying languages or other subjects and anxious to supplement their income with some occasional work. However, do not expect this to be cheap as you are likely to have to pay the full commercial rate for one-to-one instruction. You may have some friends who are prepared to make up a small class and so reduce the cost. It is advisable to insist on a systematic programme with this method, or the instruction may be haphazard or prolonged interminably.

If it is inevitable that you must delay any language instruction until after your arrival in the new country and the above methods are not open to you then there is one more alternative to consider. Very likely there are local people who want to learn your language for commercial or other reasons just as much as you want to learn their tongue. You can turn this to your mutual advantage by teaching one another at no cost. Ideally both students should be at approximately the same level, whether this is advanced, intermediate or elementary. Although not essential, similarity of age group or interests is an additional bonus. In my opinion this form of leaning is best organized into a series of role playing dialogues on various topics, which are given in one language and then repeated in the other. Whichever way you decide to learn the language then please do it systematically. Those people who say they will gradually 'pick it up as they go along' seldom reach the stage of being able to string even a simple sentence together.

Finally, we come to the matter of regional dialects which are found in various parts of many countries. In my opinion there is seldom any justification for learning a dialect, as in the vast majority of cases the main language of the country is generally understood in parallel and you should not have any difficulty in making yourself understood. If you research the reasons for the development of a dialect you almost invariably find that it arose originally due to the difficulty of communications, particularly in mountainous areas. As contacts improve in the modern world my opinion is that dialects will gradually die out. Of course, there will be local political initiative and pressure groups to attempt to keep dialects alive, but I think that they will be fighting a losing battle. For those expatriates who have children of school age and there is a choice of educational establishments teaching either the main language or a dialect, then I would advise against the latter for the reasons given above. For example, in eastern Spain there are schools teaching in Valenciano, Alicantino, Lemsin and Murciano. Apart from seeing them on bi-lingual signposts and a few official forms, they are not used very much except for speech in the villages and countryside.

10 Pensions

The rules for entitlement to a state retirement pension vary between countries and the regulations are almost invariably available in leaflet form, and there is always advice from the relevant office. In the UK the rules regarding entitlement to a retirement pension are contained in leaflet NP 32 and the current rates are listed in NI 196. A free telephone enquiry service, Freeline Social Security, can be contacted by dialling 0800-666555. If you are a British expatriate then you should deal with the Department of Social Security, Overseas Branch, Newcastle-upon-Tyne NE98 1YX, England; although if you only require the regulations they are probably obtainable much more quickly by writing to Leaflets Unit, PO Box 21, Stanmore, Middlesex HA7 1AY. Other relevant publications are NI 38 Social Security Abroad and SA 29 Your social security, health care and pension rights in the European Community, as well as separate leaflets for each country with which the UK has reciprocal arrangements for social security.

There is therefore no point in reproducing the regulations here and so the best service which I can provide is to explain some of the more complicated and unexpected points. In the latter category many readers may be surprised to learn that it is not necessary to have paid contributions for every week up to retiring age. Providing that you have made contributions for at least 90 per cent of your working life you are likely to receive a full pension. Even if you do not qualify for the latter, providing that you have paid contributions for a minimum of seven to ten years (depending upon the length of your working life), then you will be given a proportionally reduced pension. At any time before reaching retirement age you can contact your local Social Security office to discover whether you are likely to qualify for a full pension. If not and you are short of just a few stamps in a year it is well worth paying the small amount involved to make that a qualifying year. However, it is doubtful whether your best interests would be served by paying a full year's voluntary contributions to obtain an uplift of about 2.5 per cent in your pension rate, as you may well have to live four or five years from retirement age before you even begin to recoup the outlay. Probably you would be better advised to invest the sum involved, as the return would be immediate and the capital sum would pass to your heirs rather than being lost to the state on your death.

A man reaches retirement age at sixty-five and a woman at sixty in the UK. A wife can qualify for her own pension at the latter age through her own full contributions, but not on married women's reduced rate contributions. At sixty-five a man is entitled to an increased benefit for a wife, whatever her age. In addition to the basic pension you may also receive a graduated pension for such contributions paid between 1961 and 1975; as well as an additional pension under the State Earnings Related Pension Scheme based on your earnings since April 1978. You should apply for your pension three to four months before reaching the relevant age, requesting the necessary form from your Social Security office if one is not sent to you automatically.

If your retirement abroad is partial or of a transient nature you can allow your pension to accumulate for up to three months and draw it upon your return to Britain. At present the UK has reciprocal social security agreements with the following states:

Australia	Guernsey	Mauritius
Austria	Iceland	Netherlands
Belgium	Ireland	New Zealand
Bermuda	Italy	Norway
Canada	Isle of Man	Portugal
Cyprus	Israel	Spain
Denmark	Jamaica	Switzerland
Finland	Jersey	Turkey
France	Luxembourg	USA
Germany	Malta	Yugoslavia

You can receive your British retirement pension in any of the above. Even where there is no such agreement the Department of Social Security can usually arrange for payment of your pension in most countries of the world. In any case you can have it paid into a bank account and then arrange transfer abroad.

The reciprocal agreements in most, but not all, cases cover the annual uplifting of pension rates to take account of UK inflation. The exceptions are Australia, Canada, New Zealand and Norway, where you will continue to receive the pension only at the rate originally granted. This is a very serious problem for those who rely on their pension to provide all or a substantial part of their income. The annual rate of inflation in Australia recently was 8.6 per cent, so that in just four years you would lose one third of your purchasing power and in six years over half. You also need to remember that the increase covers only UK inflation and if the rate is higher in your country of retirement then you will need to fund the difference. For instance, during the past decade inflation has reached 25 per cent in Spain at times when British inflation has been much lower. You also need to consider reduction in the value of sterling against other currencies, as it has depreciated by 16 per cent against the Spanish peseta during a recent year. For the above and other reasons it is essential to have investments denominated in a variety of currencies and offshore funds are ideal for this purpose.

Occupational pension schemes vary enormously, because each one is tailored to meet the specific requirements of an individual company or group. Most schemes are reputed to be 'inflation-proof' although this may not be literally true, even for British residents. A recent survey by R. Watson & Sons, leading consulting actuaries, found that in the year to January 1989, company pensions showed an average rise of 4.7 per cent during a time when the British Retail Price Index increased by 6.8 per cent, so that rises were only 69 per cent of inflation. Even though there were often substantial surpluses in many funds these were shared between increased pensions and contribution-free periods for employees. Remember that the schemes are jointly owned by the employers and employees. Consequently you are entitled to information regarding the finances of the scheme and if you want to learn more about its operation then contact the company secretary (or other executive who deals with this matter) or the trustees. If you are not satisfied with the present policy regarding increases for inflation then complain to your trade union or to the trustees. Again, private pension schemes are also very variable, because they are designed by individual insurance companies. You will need to study the documents in your possession to form an opinion on whether this pension provides adequate protection against inflation in your country of residence. Remember that in some countries inflation may not be in single figures and it can be thousands per cent per annum.

Now we come to the question of taxation of pensions and obviously I cannot give you this information for every country in the world. All I can do in the space available is to give, by way of a single example, the taxation position for the British expatriate on pensions emanating from the UK. Obviously, all types of pensions will be assessable in your country of residence as income, without exception. Similarly all pensions, as for other incomes, arising in the UK are subject to British tax. By concession the Inland Revenue authorities in the UK allow British state retirement pensions to be paid gross. This concession does not extend to occupational and private pensions. These will be paid net after deduction of UK income tax unless you live in a country which has a Double Taxation Treaty with the UK and you complete the necessary application for gross payment, have it stamped by the revenue authorities in your country of residence and forward it to H.M. Inspector of Foreign Dividends, Lynwood road, Thames Ditton, Surrey KT7 0DP. Occupational pensions emanating from state or local government sources, such as to former members of the armed services, civil servants, teachers, police, etc., are always paid net after deduction of UK tax and can never be paid gross. However, remember that since 6th April 1990, a British subject living abroad can now claim the full UK personal allowance against income tax without reference to or disclosure of global income. A point to bear in mind is that such a claim for UK personal allowance brings into tax interest on deposits with building societies and banks which you are receiving gross as a result of self-certification of non-UK residence. In such circumstances it makes sense to move these funds to the Channel Islands, Isle of Man, or other offshore location.

11 Documentation

An aspect of expatriate life which nobody enjoys is the bureaucracy. Obviously every country has to keep track of the foreigners who come to live there, although the records in many cases may seem excessive and certain countries such as India have turned bureaucracy into an art form. Nevertheless, however tedious or demanding the regulations are it is important, as I have stressed earlier, to comply with them; even if for no other reason than peace of mind. In most foreign countries the law allows the police to eject you at very short notice with insufficient time to rearrange your affairs if you fail to comply with immigration regulations; quite apart from the likelihood of a substantial fine for breaking the law.

If you want to live in a foreign country the first step is to obtain a visa. In many cases, such as Spain and Portugal for instance, this visa can only be obtained in your home country before departure and not after arrival abroad. Therefore you should contact the embassy or consulate of the state concerned to discover the current regulations. Visas should be obtained shortly before your departure as they invariably have a time limit.

For the latter reason it is important to start collecting together the various documents you will need to produce in order to obtain a residence permit as quickly as possible, because it can take a considerable amount of time before you are in possession of all of them. The one which often takes longest is the confirmation of income and so it is imperative to arrange at an early stage for funds to be transferred to your intended country of residence on a regular monthly basis. If the combination of the bureaucracy and a foreign language which you do not understand proves too much, it is usually possible to engage a legal executive or a local agent to handle the work of obtaining a residence permit on payment of a small fee. A residence permit does not change your nationality: it merely allows you to remain in the country for a stated length of time; after which it will require renewal.

An International Driving Licence normally allows you to drive for a limited period in most foreign countries. This licence is intended for short stay visitors and it is seldom accepted on a long term basis. It is your responsibility to discover the current regulations regarding driving licences in your country of residence as ignorance of the law is no excuse for failing to have the correct documents. In many states it is a requirement when driving to carry your licence, other vehicle documents and insurance details, as well as your passport, at all times. Failure to do so can result in an immediate fine. Although the new British pink driving licence is marked 'EC' on the front cover, countries such as Spain do not recognize it as being valid for permanent residents. Foreign licences can be used up to a year in Spain, but if you intend to remain permanently in that country then you need a Spanish driving licence.

Many states have been discovering in recent years that they are losing a considerable amount of revenue due to expatriates evading taxes which they are due to pay. The lax attitude of the past is now changing rapidly, particularly with the advent of computerization. To facilitate this, control registration for a fiscal identification number is being introduced in conjunction with or separately from obtaining a residence permit. Often banking transactions are only possible upon production of this number.

The above is not necessarily an exhaustive list of all the documentation you will need in every country and you should make local enquiries from the relevant authorities.

12   Removal

It is fairly rare for someone to retire abroad and take all their worldly possessions with them on an aircraft or in their car. Although I did once travel with a Brazilian family who were setting up a new home in the Amazon jungle, taking an enormous pile of luggage on the bus with them. We travelled for five days and nights, thousands of miles across the remote Mato Grosso, along unsurfaced tracks and sometimes virgin bush when tropical rains made the route axle deep in mud. Of course, they were not popular with the other passengers on the frequent occasions when we had to pile out and push the bus because it was stuck in the mud.

Let me warn you right away that a great many expatriates suffer anguish in connection with the removal of their possessions abroad. Often many of the problems are related to the inexperience of overseas removals and ignorance of customs procedures by the removal firms concerned. At Khartoum airport when I worked for the League of Red Cross Societies in the Sudan I saw massive compounds of goods which had been uncleared for years, as customs procedures required eighty-three separate operations all to be performed in the correct sequence. Although much of this was food and aid destined for starving and destitute refugees, many organizations had given up the struggle to find a way through the labyrinth of bureaucracy. In Spain a Swedish friend of mine went every day for seven weeks to the customs post to clear his effects, only to be told each time '*mañana*' (tomorrow). These are not isolated incidents and customs regulations are very strictly imposed. In some countries outside Europe the officials are extremely corrupt and if they appear deliberately obstructive then they may be looking for a bribe to smooth the way. Some people will be totally against furthering this misuse of official power. Others may reluctantly play along as the only means of unlocking an impasse. If you decide to follow the latter course you should not make an outright offer of money, but proceed with circumspection; such as handing over your passport containing a banknote which you had 'forgotten' was there, or 'accidentally' on purpose leaving a carton of cigarettes on the desk of the customs chief.

It is very easy to find advertisements for firms offering removals abroad, although you should not make your selection on the basis of eye-catching publicity. If at all possible it is advisable to make enquiries from expatriates in your country of destination, asking them which companies they used and whether the service was satisfactory. Charges can vary enormously between different firms for an identical journey and it is advisable to draw up a short list of about five possibilities and ask for quotations. Make certain that they are offering a door-to-door service, as considerable extra costs can be involved if they are only making delivery into a customs warehouse.

Where the removal company is familiar with the customs procedures they will handle the documentation in a professional manner and the only information which they are likely to need from you is a complete list of contents of the various packages, unless they have also done the packing. If you are putting effects into store temporarily it is important therefore to prepare a list of contents before doing so, because you may not have access for this purpose later. Many countries ask for a substantial sum as a customs bond in connection with such importations. Thousands of pounds may be demanded for which you have not budgeted and the money may be held for years earning no interest and depreciating in value through inflation. Consequently, it is very important to make careful enquiries on this subject from official sources (not inaccurate gossip) before arranging importation. For instance, some countries allow your effects in duty free providing that you hold, or have applied for, a residence permit. In such circumstances it is worth considering whether you can manage without these things for a while and pay minimal storage charges at home until you have the necessary status. Those people who are arranging the importation themselves should certainly visit the appropriate consulate in their country of origin at the earliest opportunity, as contents lists will need to be stamped and there may well be other formalities. If clearance through customs could prove difficult for you, a good customs agent can save time. The better ones are respected professional organizations; but be warned that there are others on the fringe who are little more than confidence tricksters. If you engage an agent have a clear quotation for the work, pay only official disbursements against receipts and settle the fee after you have received your goods.

It is very important to ensure that your possessions are covered by insurance against all relevant risks throughout every stage of their journey. Firstly, check your insurance policy in your home country if it is still in force to see what cover it continues to provide. Quite likely the removal company will include insurance cover in their quotation, as they receive commission from the insurers. You may well consider that the charge is reasonable and this is a convenient arrangement. However, remember that you are under no obligation to accept both removal charge and insurance quotation if the latter seems excessive. You are at liberty to arrange your own insurance if you can find better cover at a lower premium, providing that you make it clear to the removal firm that you do not require their insurance. Also bear in mind that immediately on arrival of your goods the value of contents in your new house increases substantially and you will want to increase the cover for contents without delay. Thieves are often on the watch for the arrival of valuable articles and this is a favourite time for a break-in.

People often get very attached to furniture which they have had for years and they hate to see it go for next to nothing when they had to work hard to buy it originally. Nevertheless, if you are moving abroad then this is the time for a dispassionate look at practicalities. Removal of furniture abroad can seldom be justified on economic grounds, because the weight and bulk makes transport costs extremely expensive. In most cases you would be well advised to sell the old furniture for whatever it will fetch and to save the high removal costs towards the purchase of new items. In any case, the latter bought locally are much more likely to be better suited to the changed conditions to be found in your country of retirement. Naturally, antiques are a different matter and they merit special consideration, providing that they are likely to stand up to changed weather conditions, such as higher temperatures and possibly greater humidity. The final word must be to plan your removal well, or you could be in for a traumatic time.

13   Settling In

You may well think that all you have to do is to move abroad and you can sit back and relax for the remainder of your life – well not quite! Firstly, there are a number of essential matters which you need to attend to, which are likely to take months or perhaps up to a year. So before you spend all your time sunbathing on the beach or sipping cool drinks on your verandah get these jobs out of the way. If you leave them there will be a guilty conscience detracting from your enjoyment of your retirement and in the case of certain serious delays you could be forced to leave and return home. There is no need to go to the other extreme like one couple I know, who said they were thinking of returning after a week because they had not obtained a residence permit. Such matters take time in a foreign country and it is important not to panic but to work steadily and systematically through the various items as opportunity allows. In this connection it is often helpful to prepare a priority list enumerating the various matters in sequence or urgency. For those of you who think that they will have nothing to do, how about opening local bank accounts, completing the purchase of your property, arranging house and contents insurance, buying furniture, paying electricity and water connection charges, plus gas if required, registering with the local health service, arranging private medical insurance if desired, commencing transfers for living expenses, applying for a residence permit, hiring or purchasing a car, obtaining a local driving licence, registering with your consul, learning the language, arranging removal of your effects plus insurance, registering your deeds, engaging a financial consultant, moving your assets offshore, registering with the local fiscal authorities, completing tax returns, making a will, obtaining a pet, building an extension to your property if desired, or a patio or swimming pool, fencing the plot, planning and planting the garden, joining clubs and evaluating television services?

In Appendix I of this book I have given a typical expatriate checklist. This can only be a generalization because both items and timing will vary between different countries and for individual people. However, it may help to jog your memory regarding some essential matters. You will see that I have given an earliest and a latest date for each matter which you will need to adjust to the particular circumstances in your country of residence. Some items may be of rather less importance and you can think about them for a year or two before making a decision. Others may have very strict time limits, such as applying for a residence permit, and you will need to give these your urgent attention, otherwise you may well have to return to your country of origin for a fresh visa because the original one is out of date. You can prepare your own individual priority list by listing items in order of latest dates for completion.

Obviously you will want to be on friendly terms with your new neighbours, if for no other reason than the alternative is likely to lead to continuous tensions. If problems are encountered living alongside other people then they are best solved by a friendly and amicable discussion, as your neighbours may be quite unaware that they are causing you an annoyance. The wrong response is to use argument, threats and retaliation, as these are likely to prove counter-productive and lead to an escalation in tension. As regards other friendships, it is probably good advice to build these up gradually and steadily rather than rush into them too quickly. If you don't you may well find the pattern of your lifestyle being dictated to you instead of being of your own choosing, as you are saddled with the person who has been starved of company and wants to spend all day in your house talking. One unfortunate aspect of expatriate life is that people often form themselves into cliques and it is better to take your time about deciding whether you really want to join them. You may not be meeting just one new nationality, but in a cosmopolitan area there may be many. People of every state have different customs and taboos, so it is advisable to attempt to learn about these as soon as possible to avoid causing unintentional offence to your hosts.

Clubs and societies of some kind or other are very likely to be open to you (unless you move to a very isolated area) and again my advice is not to rush into membership, but to see how the group activities could fit into your overall pattern of living. Very often they accept people as guests without actually joining and this is a good introduction. If your means are limited you may need to consider how the costs are likely to relate to your budget. For instance, golf is frequently very expensive abroad and it can be extremely embarrassing to be asked to play much more often than you can afford. Similarly, you should give the matter very careful consideration if you are invited to become an official of a club or society as this can be very demanding of your time.

14   Culture Shock

Culture shock is what most people suffer to greater or lesser extent when going abroad, even for a short holiday. The less experience a person has of conditions outside his or her own country then the more likelihood there is of being affected to a higher level. One of the strangest aspects of this condition is that most people do not even realize that they are suffering from culture shock.

How does it manifest itself? It arises because various countries present differences, which may be profound, in living conditions, eating habits, social contact, infrastructure development, administrative procedures, routines, climate, honesty, public accountability and one hundred and one other matters which affect everyday life. In short, as many people say, 'It is not like back home.'

Make no mistake about it, culture shock needs recognition and self-treatment or a chronic medical condition can easily result, with possibly the only cure being the expensive one of selling your new property and returning to your original country. How do you recognize culture shock? Well, the sentence at the end of the previous paragraph, or a close variant of it, is a sure sign. Naturally, anyone on first arrival in a new country will note the novel features. Culture shock can easily be diagnosed when after this initial period you continue to make comparisons with your country of origin, particularly only on adverse matters.

The vast majority of people are very resistant to change and this is particularly true of the higher age groups who have reached retirement. To counter culture shock it is very important to adopt a positive attitude and give due consideration to the advantages of retirement abroad, such as dry warm weather, lower fuel costs and taxes, etc., which you tend to take for granted and forget; rather than to latch on to only the unfavourable comparisons. The circle of friends which you choose can have a very marked effect upon your own enjoyment of retirement abroad. If this consists mainly of people who complain and denigrate the institutions and customs of the new country all day then you will be subjected to a continual brainwashing which will also make you unhappy. Avoid such people – or better still, help them over their culture shock by encouraging them to adopt positive attitudes in place of their negative ones.

Life in a new country may mean that you need to adopt different routines to those of where you originated. In Spain the afternoon rest during siesta is almost a national institution and there would be a general outcry if the government suggested changing it. You may well say, 'I've never gone to bed in the afternoon in my life and I don't intend to start now.' Even so, it makes sense to relax on a sunbed after lunch, perhaps doing some reading. To carry on gardening or some other physical work in the sun during the heat of the day is likely to lead to sunstroke. Quite apart from the fact that global warming has resulted in the climate becoming progressively hotter, this has been recognized since Noël Coward's day, so take notice of the lyrics of his song:

> In tropical climes there are certain times of day
> When all the citizens retire
> To tear their clothes off and perspire.
> It's one of those rules that the greatest fools obey,
> Because the sun is much too sultry
> And one must avoid its ultry-violet ray ...

> Mad dogs and Englishmen
> Go out in the midday sun,
> The Japanese don't care to
> The Chinese wouldn't dare to,
> Hindoos and Argentines sleep firmly from twelve to one.
> But Englishmen detest a siesta.
> In the Philippines
> There are lovely screens
> To protect you from the glare.
> In the Malay States
> There are hats like plates
> Which the Britishers won't wear.
> At twelve noon

The natives swoon
And no further work is done.
But mad dogs and Englishmen
Go out in the midday sun.

It's such a surprise for the Eastern eyes to see
That though the English are effete,
They're quite impervious to heat,
When the white man rides every native hides in glee,
Because the simple creatures hope he
Will impale his solar topee on a tree …

Mad dogs and Englishmen
Go out in the midday sun.
The toughest Burmese bandit
Can never understand it.
In Rangoon the heat of noon
Is just what the natives shun.
They put their Scotch or Rye down
And lie down.
In a jungle town
Where the sun beats down
To the rage of man and beast
The English garb
Of the English sahib
Merely gets a bit more creased.

In Bangkok
At twelve o'clock
They foam at the mouth and run,
But mad dogs and Englishmen
Go out in the midday sun.

Mad dogs and Englishmen
Go out in the midday sun.
The smallest Malay rabbit
Deplores this stupid habit.
In Hong Kong
They strike a gong
And fire off a noonday gun
To reprimand each inmate
Who's in late.
In the mangrove swamps
Where the python romps
There is no peace from twelve till two.

Even caribous
Lie around and snooze,
For there's nothing else to do.
In Bengal
To move at all
Is seldom, if ever done,
But mad dogs and Englishmen
Go out in the midday sun.

Do not repeat the mistake which many Americans make abroad by saying to the local people, 'You do things the wrong way', rather than the more accurate, 'You do things a different way from us'. These local people have traditions and experience extending over thousands of years and it is dismissive to imply that their knowledge of local conditions counts for nothing. Certainly new technologies, such as have produced air-conditioning units for instance, can effect changes. This consideration apart, you have to accept the local situation as it is and embrace the country warts and all if you are going to live there. One person cannot change the state, its institutions and the whole of its population. To attempt to do so is equivalent to banging you head against a brick wall and the effort will just make you unhappy without having the slightest effect upon change. So live the local life – don't fight it. How will you know when you are winning your battle against culture shock? When you stop converting local prices into the currency of your homeland.

15 Transportation

If you are going to live abroad then transportation will be an important consideration as you are unlikely to spend all of your time in one place, because it would be boring to do so. There may be certain reasons why you will not own a car, such as not having a driving licence or being unable to hold one due to infirmity, besides the possibility that your budget will not run to the costs involved. Fortunately, the days of the memsahib are passing and so are the objections to travelling with 'the natives'. In a large number of countries abroad the standard of public transport is acceptable, although women travelling alone may be subject to harassment in places such as Italy and many Arab states. Also it can be quite a fight to board a vehicle on busy services, even in civilized countries such as France. In many parts of the world queuing in line is not followed and a free-for-all scramble takes place. This still leaves quite a number of areas where public transport is excessively hot, uncomfortable, overcrowded, dirty, poorly maintained and erratic. So if you are going to have to depend upon public transport it is important to check that it is satisfactory and acceptable. In most resort areas out of season the service may be sparse or non-existent. It may surprise many of you to learn that in a lot of countries travel by railway is cheaper than by bus, although the trains are often slow and follow a circuitous route. Unfortunately, due to rising fuel prices the number of places where taxis can be used regularly at low cost is rapidly shrinking. Collective taxis are more economical where they are an institution, such as in Turkey, the Andean countries and other parts of Latin America.

The cost of car hire on a long term basis can seldom be justified on economic grounds; although it may be a useful stopgap, such as when evaluating the local motor car market rather than rushing into a hurried and unwise purchase. Shop around regarding rates, as the international companies tend to be expensive and you may well find local firms offering an identical car and equivalent service at a much lower cost.

Importing a vehicle into a foreign country involves two separate considerations. Firstly, whether it is worth your while to bring in a car which you have used in your original homeland. The customs duty is likely to vary according to the age of the vehicle and it can be quite low on an older model. However, if it is a right-hand drive car from Britain my advice is to sell it before emigration, as it is dangerous to overtake with such a vehicle in countries where they drive on the right. Spain now bars such permanent importations. Secondly, there is the possibility of importing a new model from places such as Andorra, Gilbraltar or Denmark where there is little or no vehicle duty. I cannot generalize about whether this is advantageous as it depends upon the local regulations in your country of residence, which you will need to check. In either case, even if no customs duty is payable, you must remember that rates of value added tax can vary enormously between different states and a substantial sum could be payable on this account. For example, the rate of VAT on cars in Britain was 15 per cent and in Spain it was 33 per cent. Therefore, if you imported a vehicle from the UK into Spain you used to have to pay the differential of 18 per cent of its value.

Assuming that importation does not confer any special benefits then you will probably decide upon a local purchase. It is a good idea to discover which are the popular makes of car in your retirement country as mechanics will be familiar with these models and parts will be readily available. If you go outside this range, in the absence of a local dealer, service could be poor and the availability of parts subject to long delays. In many Third World states they just do not have the necessary foreign exchange available to import foreign cars and parts. You may be surprised to learn that in Uruguay the vast majority of the few cars to be seen are Ford Model T's of the 1930s, even in smart resorts such as Punta del Este.

If you are buying a new car you do not necessarily have to pay the list price. Make enquiries in the local area to discover what promotional discounts are on offer. It may well be possible to buy a new car at fleet price if you search around for the right contacts. Organizations purchasing about twenty or more vehicles at a time, such as car hire companies, can easily add one extra and there is often a fair amount of choice. Usually they are satisfied with the commission involved as their margin on the deal.

Buying a used car in a foreign country is fraught with potential hazards. Do not assume that the legal protection for purchasers in your home country necessarily applies abroad because in the latter you are frequently buying a car 'as seen'. Sometimes guarantees are given and you can find that these are practically worthless. Always insist that a guarantee is given in writing. Even so, it will often cover parts only and you would find it difficult to dispute whatever charge is made for labour, particularly as the dealer is likely to insist that a garage of his choice is used for service. For these and other reasons it is essential to get to know the local second-hand car market reasonably well before you buy. Certainly make enquiries from your fellow expatriates regarding their experiences and ask for their recommendations, although beware of those who act as agents on commission. If you do not have a very high level of mechanical knowledge it is worthwhile taking an experienced person with you when buying a second-hand car, even if you have to pay a fee, as the important point is what is under the bonnet and not particularly the appearance of the bodywork. Remember also that climatic conditions differ between countries and that this can have a considerable effect upon the average life of a vehicle. For instance, in southern Europe many areas are permanently free of snow and ice so that no salt is used on the roads, leading to very little rust of the chassis. Also the upper portion does not deteriorate so quickly in the dry atmosphere. As a result some car dealers may be inclined to understate the age of the vehicle by a considerable amount, so it is advisable to ask to see the relevant papers.

Which brings us to the matter of documentation. It is important to familiarize yourself with the current requirements regarding vehicle documents in your country of residence. Always insist on receiving all of the papers on completion of a purchase and refuse to hand over the balance of the price on promises to supply them later. Without these documents it may well prove impossible to register the car in your name or to put it through obligatory vehicle tests. It is your responsibility to discover when periodical inspections are due. You should also take local advice on how to protect yourself from the possibility of buying a vehicle subject to a hire purchase agreement on which outstanding sums may be due. Make certain that the road fund tax has been paid up to date, or you could find yourself due to pay for past years. Always keep the documentation in order and carry the papers whenever driving if this is the local law. Never buy a former hire car, as after one year it is likely to be in an equivalent mechanical state as a car in private ownership for ten years. Again the documents should show this, as the former owner is likely to be a company. The final word must be to discover the reputation of dealers and how much attention they pay to the points enumerated above.

16   Food and Drink

Most people's expenditure on the food which they buy to prepare themselves does not differ a great deal within a particular country. The big variable is how often you eat out and so, if this is likely to be frequently, it is advisable to confirm that restaurant meals will be within your budget. Special deals are often on offer, which can be a menu of the day with a certain amount of choice. Such promotions tend to be found more often during the day than in the evening. Consider the price of meals in restaurants in relation to the local costs of the ingredients and you may well find that some are not good value. For instance, quite high charges may be made for salads, which you could very easily prepare yourself for a small fraction of the charge. For those of you to whom inexpensive restaurants are an important consideration in the selection of a retirement home I could mention Mexico, where I had an eight course meal in 1986 in Guadalajara for one US dollar; or even better, Bolivia where in 1982 in Santa Cruz I enjoyed a three course meal with steak and eggs for the equivalent of just eight pence sterling.

Whether you go to restaurants or stick to your own cooking, do be adventurous and sample some of the local dishes. They tend to use produce which is plentiful and cheap, as well as being dishes which are often suited to the climate. The latter could be in doubt if you try the local curry in the Seychelles Islands, where you may be tempted to call the brigade to put out the fire in your mouth, which lasts long after the meal. Highly spiced dishes are best approached gradually and with care, as they can easily cause digestive problems for the uninitiated. Of course, there will be some local dishes which will fill you with revulsion, whether it is snails in France or roast guinea-pig in Peru and no amount of coaxing from the residents will induce you to try them.

Shopping is always a new experience in a different country. The main problem is likely to be that local people are charged one price and expatriates a much higher one. The latter have only themselves to blame for this situation, as visitors tend to pay whatever is asked without question and to regard the local currency as 'Mickey Mouse money', not having any real value. Shops situated in areas with a fairly high proportion of foreign residents tend to be the ones which charge inflated prices. If you go to those in districts peopled by nationals then you are likely to find that prices are much lower. Of course, the former tend to be the only ones which stock items familiar to you back home and if you want them then you will have to pay the high charges of importation. The main way of overcoming this differential pricing problem is to do most of your shopping at supermarkets and similar establishments where prices are fixed and displayed. Even these situated in resort areas will tend to push up many prices during the holiday season. Most people abroad are far too trusting and lose considerable sums through being short-changed, without ever realizing it. Due to unfamiliarity with the language they are often unsure how much is being asked and tender a high value note. Be particularly careful of these slick operators who quickly hand you the coins, pausing a long time before looking for small notes and even longer before finding larger notes, hoping that you will walk away during the intervals assuming that you have been given all your change. So focus your attention on the notes and not the coins.

Covered and open air markets almost invariably tend to be good value for fruit and vegetables. This may also be the case for such items as meat, fish, dairy produce or even general groceries, as overheads are less than for a shop. You are likely to find much better value in a quiet country area than in one where a large number of tourists shop. In the latter many items can be dearer in a market than in a high class department store, as foreigners do not know local prices well enough. In times of high yields for fruit and vegetables you are likely to obtain the benefit of very low prices. This is because the stall holders are often also the growers and they want to dispose of all of the crop quickly for what it will fetch, rather than transport unsold stock back to their farm where there may be unsuitable and inadequate storing facilities. Remember that markets are a favourite hunting ground for skilled pickpockets in many countries. Never engage in gambling games in a market.

Alcohol comes in a great many shapes and forms. Quite likely the whole spectrum will be available in your country of retirement at considerably less cost than back home, where the price is inflated by customs and excise duties. As a result, quite a few expatriates tend to consume a very excessive amount of alcohol. In a hot climate you should drink at least six to eight pints of some liquid each day. The mistake which many make is to have this intake solely in the form of alcoholic drinks. The result is often a progressive state of alcoholism which, if not corrected, can easily be (and often is) fatal. It is a widespread problem and there are self-help organizations in many areas. Having said that, there is no reason why you should not enjoy wine, beer or the occasional glass of spirits in moderation, as there is no medical evidence that this is unhealthy.

Soft drinks come in a similar dazzling array of choices, some of which may be unfamiliar to you and others being well-known brands produced locally under licence. The latter have their international reputation to protect and the former may be just as safe and pleasing to drink. In the vast majority of countries all such drinks are manufactured and bottled under controlled conditions. Beware that in parts of Latin America and elsewhere you may not be drinking what you think you are consuming if it is in a bottle with a cap which can be pressed back on again after filling with some alternative liquid. Such operators tend to be active around public transport terminals where passengers are desperate for a drink. It may be a matter of doubt whether the bottles or the contents are the more unhygienic. Cans are far safer.

In countries where there is the slightest doubt about the advisability of drinking the water you should have precisely the same reservations regarding ice. Freezing does not kill germs; only boiling water normally does that. You should assume, in the absence of incontrovertible evidence to the contrary, that practically all ice served in public places is produced from untreated tap water and this can well also be the case in multi-stellar hotels. In areas where bilharzia is prevalent, which includes practically the whole of Africa, the public water supply should be filtered as well as boiled before being consumed in any form, including ice. Of course, you will make your own decision based on local conditions whether you rely entirely on bottled water.

17 Entertainment

Entertainment possibilities will vary enormously between different countries and you should check that there will be sufficient available locally to keep you amused. Perhaps you will be able to dress up and go to a casino. Many states do not allow their own nationals to enter casinos, which are restricted to foreigners; so in such cases you will need to carry your passport. A number of casinos are expanding slot machine facilities to a wider clientele, however they are dressed.

Nightclubs also come in a vast array of types, from sleazy dives to establishments of top class entertainment. Do not have regard only to the appearance of the building, as you can frequently find superb jazz played in a cellar and tourist rip off rubbish staged in a large auditorium. Be careful of what you are getting yourself into as, for instance, in Spain a nightclub alongside a main highway is often a euphemism for a brothel.

Parks, likewise, come in many different forms. Almost every country has amusement parks, although the question of whether you are likely to enjoy the razzle-dazzle of such places is quite another matter. 'Aquaparks' are being set up in a number of the warmer resort areas, but these are likely to appeal more to younger people and those with children. Safari parks have seen a similar proliferation. The wide open spaces could appeal to you even if you do not like to see animals caged in a zoo. Always take your opportunities to visit botanical gardens, whether they are superb as in Rio de Janeiro or more modest local ones, because they can tell you a great deal about the indigenous flora. Even if the park is just a municipal one it may be well maintained and this is an ideal place to meet and converse with local people on a seat under the shade of a tree.

In many places the folklore is extremely rich in the history of the country besides being lavishly costumed in the traditional dress, and you do not necessarily have to be proficient in the language to appreciate the spectacle. It would be a pity to miss any such events through lack of advance information, so it is best to check with your local tourist office regarding regional attractions, as they normally know the dates well in advance.

Just about every country in the world has international clubs, British clubs, country clubs and many others where entry may be open or restricted. Sometimes they centre their activities on a single sport and others provide a wide gambit of interests from bingo to bridge. Often members are able to sign in guests and if you have a friend who is a member then this is a good way to discover whether the club is likely to appeal to you without committing yourself. Where accommodation is very limited and new members are only accepted as vacancies occur it is a good idea to apply for membership and join the waiting list at the earliest opportunity, as you can usually withdraw your application if you change your mind in the interim before being offered membership. In the past many such clubs often had a colonial mentality, but fortunately this is now changing for the better.

Most, but not all, countries have seen a demise in cinemas as a result of competition from television. Some resurgence is just detectable and it is certainly true that many films shot on location are far more enjoyable when seen on a wide screen rather than on a small box. Standards of comfort will vary a great deal between countries. In a hot climate you may have open-air cinemas or air-conditioning. With greater seasonal differences a sliding roof could be incorporated into the structure. The film may be made in the local language, or it may be foreign produced and dubbed or sub-titled. Whichever it is, films are a very effective way of learning a language and picking up the colloquial expressions. So if it is a movie which depends rather more on its action than its dialogue then it should not detract too much from your enjoyment, even if you are not fluent in the local language. One thing is certain – you will understand more each time you go.

Language is much more of a problem where theatres are concerned, as the entertainment is centred upon the enjoyment of dialogue, modes of speech and the nuances of expression. Even so, there are many musical productions where you can enjoy the orchestra, the songs and the dances with little or no knowledge of the language. Anyway, if theatre is your passion why not stage amateur productions with your friends?

Just because you are a long way from your homeland it does not necessarily follow that you are in a cultural wilderness. More than a hundred years ago, long before the advent of air travel, complete top companies from Europe performed operas and plays in Manaus, 1,000 miles up the Amazon river. Today you can see the very best international class ballets, operas, concerts and other productions in Rio de Janeiro on a continuous basis. Superb opera is always available in many Italian cities. Bear in mind also that theatre and other companies with the highest reputations frequently go on tour abroad, so look out for likely venues. You would well see an identical production locally at a small fraction of the cost in London. In any event, concerts have no linguistic barriers and they are widely performed.

18 Sports and Pastimes

Television standards have fallen so dramatically in recent years that it probably does not deserve the appellation of entertainment and it is relegated to a pastime which you sometimes follow when you have nothing else to do. Even the previously excellent BBC is no exception, following the nonsensical scramble for ratings, although it still does not carry advertising. This search for the highest common factor has resulted in standards falling to the lowest common multiple, so that its schedules are packed with rubbish and it is doubtful whether it is even complying with its charter. Most expatriates find that they watch considerably less television abroad than they did at home. There are various reasons for this. Some are glad to extricate themselves from a boring and monotonous waste of their time. Many others in a more congenial climate like to spend a lot of their leisure time on outdoor activities. Even so, television can be very useful, particularly during the longer and cooler evenings of winter months. If television in a language which you can understand is going to be a very important factor in your enjoyment of your retirement then, as mentioned in Chapter 4, it is essential to select your location with care. This is because costs can vary in different places from as little as a maintenance fee of £4 per month for cable where the appropriate wiring is part of the infrastructure, to well over £1,000 if you need to install a satellite dish.

Videos are available in a variety of languages in a great many countries and they provide a useful alternative to television if the latter programmes are not to your liking. As expatriates often have unexpected callers videos have an obvious advantage if your viewing is interrupted.

The criticisms which I have made of BBC television do not apply to the radio broadcasts of the BBC World Service, as quality is not set by the most moronic members of the population. Many of these radio programmes are informative and entertaining. *BBC Worldwide* is the programme journal of the BBC World Service, which contains the schedules for the coming month together with the recommended frequency settings for reception in all countries and regions at different times of the day or night. It is available on subscription for a small sum, or a specimen copy can be obtained free by writing to *BBC Worldwide*, PO Box 765, Bush House, Strand, London WC2B 4PH, England. You will almost certainly need a radio with at least one shortwave band and preferably two. These can be quite expensive in many foreign countries and you may be well advised to purchase a suitable radio before leaving home, as you may find some of Russian or Far Eastern manufacture at low cost. A telescopic aerial assists reception. I have found the reasonably priced Philips D-2225 very satisfactory and it contains FM, MW, and LW plus two shortwave bands. If your radio has only one SW band the preferred range to select for reception in southern Europe is 6 to 12 MHz or 24 to 48 metres. Radio amateurs will find that in most foreign countries they have to deal with a great deal of bureaucracy before they are allowed to transmit. This does not necessarily apply in the case of CB radio, which can be a fairly inexpensive hobby as well as a boon to the infirm and the lonely, particularly where telephones are non-existent.

Many retired expatriates spend a lot of time reading. Paperback books are available in the popular resort areas in a variety of languages. Frequently book exchange facilities can be used to reduce the inflated cost of importation. For more serious reading the larger bookstores in your home country are likely to have a mail order service. Some such as Waterstone & Co. Ltd of London WC2 produce a massive catalogue and publications such as *The Good Book Guide* have a bimonthly update for subscribers. The main newspapers of Europe and North America are supplied to many countries and you may find that copies are available on a regular basis. Magazines are probably better obtained on subscription if continuity of supply is important to you, due to the variability of demand and distribution abroad. At the earliest possible stage of learning the language you should attempt to read local newspapers and periodicals. You will be amazed at how quickly you can follow complete articles, besides which it will expand your vocabulary and increase your confidence.

Indoor games such as whist, bridge and chess, to mention just a few, are popular with expatriates and it should not be too difficult to find a club where they are played and tournaments held. Failing that you can always invite some friends to your house for a game.

Almost everything seems collectable these days, whether it is stamps, antiques, comics or whatever. Perhaps your hobby needs the participation of others to make it more enjoyable and practical. If so and no club exists then I can only suggest that you form one. Should your collection be valuable it is advisable to use a publication which has box numbers for replies, or you may bring your premises to the attention of prospective thieves in advertising for similar collectors.

Swimming can be followed for a long season in many warm countries, whether you prefer the sea or a pool. Sea swimming is also an inexpensive and healthy pastime. Be careful of local tidal problems and if you retire alongside the Pacific watch out for shark attacks.

Marinas are mushrooming all over the place, so that if you have the funds for a boat and the related expenses then you should not lack facilities in the popular retirement areas. Many people are buying property alongside marinas, although prices are exceptionally high. If you are only familiar with coastal sailing do remember that the Mediterranean is no lake and it can be extremely rough at times, so do not venture out without an experienced crew.

Fishing is very likely to be available, whether your property is situated on the coast or inland. However good your tackle you could draw a blank day unless you take local advice on the best locations and the correct bait to use. An inexpensive licence is frequently required. If sport fishing dominates your choice of retirement location then you may well select the Indian Ocean or the Caribbean area.

Golf courses are being built at a very rapid rate in almost every popular retirement area. If the country is a rather dry one and a great deal of expensive water is required to maintain the course in a good condition then golf is often an extremely expensive sport to follow on a regular basis. Make enquiries concerning life membership as this can be available at reasonable cost, particularly at an early stage in the development of a club. Many people buy property alongside a golf course and this often gives them free play or economical charges.

Walking and climbing are numbered amongst my favourite sports, so I could write a complete book on this subject. Due to lack of space in a book of this type I must regretfully confine myself to a few generalities. Climbing requires special conditions; but you can go walking anywhere, as I have done in places such as the Himalayas, the Central Sahara and the Andes, whether the terrain is mountains, deserts or jungles. The essentials are a large scale map, compass, clothing to protect you from wet, cold and windy weather, a tie-on hat if there is a hot sun, walking boots if the track is loose, and plenty to drink, although a person can go a long time without food. If you confine your walks to uncultivated areas you are not likely to find any obstructions or objections. It is a very healthy and inexpensive hobby in which anyone can engage. A friend of mine who is a great-grandmother never has any difficulty in getting to the top of any mountain.

Camping and caravanning also give you the opportunity of seeing the countryside in more detail at low cost. I have camped in all continents in places as far apart as northern Sweden and Uruguay, both on recognized sites and in the wild, and I have never had the slightest difficulty. Retired people with a base abroad who dislike remaining in one spot often use caravans to tour on an almost continuous basis.

As a result of heightened interest in the international tournaments, tennis has become widely available in most countries. Both private and public courts have proliferated, whether built by clubs or municipal authorities. Badminton and squash are not quite so well-known, although they are both developing.

Cycling is not widely followed except in northern Europe, although it can be very enjoyable as I found cycle-camping from Cornwall in south-west England to northern Sweden, a journey of 4,500 kilometres. Daily cycling is very healthy exercise for all, including those of retirement age, as it gets the heart pumping, which is beneficial. A bicycle can be useful to fetch the bread and small items of shopping, rather than getting the car out. Take care when cycling on the highway if roads are narrow and use the hard shoulder wherever one is available.

The availability of horse riding is very patchy and it could be confined to the popular resort areas. If you live in the countryside farmers may well be pleased to have horses exercised on an occasional basis. Keep away from roads if possible, as most drivers are unaware of the consideration which horses require on the highway.

If you wish to engage in shooting and hunting then you should choose your retirement area with great care. In the Latin countries of the Mediterranean area, shooting is reserved for the owners of the land almost everywhere, including the wilder regions. Even in many African states hunting licences are becoming expensive and difficult to obtain. The importation of firearms of all types is strictly controlled almost without exception in every country.

When moving to a retirement country most ornithologists are in for a treat regarding the sheer range of species and the colours of their plumage, quite apart from the joy of seeing many new species for the very first time. Often the feathered wildlife is very approachable. Near where I live on the Costa Blanca large groups of flamingos can frequently be seen on the salt lakes when driving past, as well as masses of wading birds and terns.

The well-known skiing centres in the various Alpine countries will be familiar to you if this is your sport. It may come as something of a surprise that skiing of a high standard could be available in a number of other locations. For instance, there is quite a long season for the sport in Spain, not only in the Pyrenees, but also in the Cantabrian mountains, near Madrid and even in the south close to Granada in the Sierra Nevada, although most people think of the country as being hot. In Morocco good skiing can be had at Mischliffen and other centres.

Self-organized keep fit classes are a feature in a large number of expatriate communities, where an indolent life and overeating wreack havoc with the waistline and other parts of the anatomy. My personal feeling is that this is a rather static and masochistic form of exercise, when the same result could be achieved in a much more enjoyable way by taking part in outdoor activities.

If I have not mentioned your particular sport it does not necessarily mean that you will not be able to follow it abroad. Some people will go to extraordinary lengths to engage in a sport. Take cricket for instance. During the Second World War a British administrator was assigned to a lonely outpost in Somaliland with no one else to play the game. He decided to use his powers as magistrate to release some criminals from jail on condition that they played cricket. After just one game they voluntarily returned to prison saying that they would rather remain locked up than play again! Brazil may seem an impossible location to find cricket, but in fact it is played regularly at Campos do Jordão between Rio de Janeiro and São Paulo.

19   Community Life

In deciding where to retire you will need to consider whether you prefer community life or wish to opt for a more isolated situation in a rural area. In coming to this decision you should think ahead to a possible changing situation in the future when you might be ill, infirm, or unable to own or drive a car. It may be possible to move if such events occur, but bear in mind the financial aspects, such as the fact that the cost of property now is higher in developed areas or may become so. Consequently, it is usually easier to move into the countryside, as this can produce surplus funds which when invested provide extra income to cope with the ravages of inflation upon your lifestyle. Conversely, elderly people of limited means who later in life need to move to where facilities are better may find it difficult to do so, because country properties can be difficult to sell and fetch less than the minimum cost of accommodation elsewhere.

Personally, I am not arguing for one situation or the other, because they both have advantages and drawbacks, so it is a question of balancing these and coming to an individual decision. One favourable aspect of community life is that it provides mutual support to ease you gradually through the culture shock of going to live in a foreign country, particularly if you are unfamiliar with the local language. When you first move in there will be a hundred and more things to be done, a process which your compatriots have been through and on which they can advise you regarding procedures. I have also found communities to be very supportive to members who encounter unexpected problems.

If you are purchasing an apartment in southern Europe the legal position in regard to parts of the building used by all the owners of flats is different from that encountered in Britain. In the UK there is usually a landlord of the freehold and apartments are purchased on a long leasehold. The landlord is normally responsible for providing common services, for which a charge is made. In the popular retirement countries of southern Europe such as Portugal, Spain, France and Italy the apartment owners have a share in the common property and bear a proportion of the cost of its upkeep, which is divided according to a legal formula. This is administered by a president elected at an annual general meeting of owners. He can be assisted by other officials, who may or may not be elected. Proxy voting by absent owners is provided for, although this can be a disadvantage in such situations as where an administrator favouring the developer collects a large number of proxies and so blocks attempts by permanent residents for improvements. The type of ownership described above does not necessarily remain restricted to apartments alone, as detached properties can be administered in the same way where there is an element of shared ownership of swimming pools, gardens, footpaths or other property. The local laws vary from country to country and further details are given in Appendix II.

In southern Europe there are many developments which are built with retired foreigners very much in mind, whether they are called urbanizations, condominiums or whatever. The properties may be purchased entirely by expatriates or there may be an element of minor or major local ownership, although these mainly tend to be holiday homes. Retired persons should be fully aware that where you have mixed ownership of permanent residents, holidaymakers and local people then they follow very different lifestyles which often clash. For instance, Spanish people usually have their evening meal about 10 p.m. so that they are quite noisy until fairly late. Vacationers mostly sleep in the sun during the day, so they are active and exuberant until 2 a.m. or after. Retired persons who want to go to bed to sleep round about 11 p.m. find this disturbance extremely stressful. If this is likely to be your reaction then, as I have impressed upon you earlier, you should choose your location with care and certainly well away from any bars or discotheques.

One of the favourable points about living in a community is that if you wish to follow an active sporting or social life then this is considerably easier to organize compared with residence in a more isolated situation. Many of the higher quality developments include a wide range of facilities. You may have an enthusiastic committee which will provide and encourage the provision of such amenities. Alternatively, you may need to take the initiative yourself and find a few like-minded people who will form the nucleus for a club to follow whichever activity interests you. Remember that these are often embryo communities and the enjoyment of the pastime will usually be proportional to the effort which you devote to its development.

20 Gardening

Some people enjoy gardening – others absolutely hate it. In between are many people who never had the time or space to engage in gardening during their working lives, but find it a very satisfying occupation to take up much of their leisure hours during retirement. When you are considering a garden you should think ahead to changes which may be desirable in the future. For instance, if you retire early you may have a very active sporting life at first, although later you may need to change this to pottering around the garden. Conversely, you could cultivate a lot of ground initially, but advancing years might mean that this becomes an unbearable burden. Thus, the point of this paragraph is to stress that before you start any gardening it is important to have a plan not only for the present but also for the future. If you go ahead quickly and have all your ground tiled then you may soon bemoan the lack of a garden. In the Mediterranean area contractors lay tiles on concrete which entails the use of a pneumatic drill to make a change. This is quite unnecessary, as tiles can be bedded firmly into sand with a rubber hammer and they will not move by as much as a millimetre even with the weight of a car upon them.

So take the measurements of your plot and commence with a scale plan. It is very much better to consider alternative positions using a pencil and rubber than to kill your plants with frequent moving. Think of the future also, because when you plant a small tree in a certain position you need to consider whether as it grows to maturity it is likely to make your house dark and cold in winter. Your objective in planning a garden should be to make it pleasing both internally from where you usually sit to view it and also externally from the eyes of people passing by. So place yourself in these positions and consider the effect. Try to avoid large expanses of tiling or gravel by breaking them up with trees or flower beds. Do not plan things such as paths in uninteresting straight lines, as curves or zigzags are much more pleasing to the eye. One aspect which your scale plan will not convey is elevation, so if the plot is rather flat consider how you can vary this with rockeries or terraced flower-beds.

Consideration should also be given to the seasons, so that you have a succession of flowering plants throughout the year; even winter being no exception in warm climates if you are bringing along in time such flowers as marigolds and pansies, for instance. If you want trees to provide shade in summer but not in winter then select decidious rather than evergreens. In Mediterranean countries the amount of growth of plants will vary enormously in shade and sunlight throughout the seasons. In summer they will make four times as much growth in the shade as in sunlight; in winter the growth is completely reversed.

Which brings us to the question of climatic variations between a person's country of origin and retirement home abroad, the latter mainly tending to be warmer and drier. Whatever these variations are, your objective should be to use them to advantage by planting the things which do well locally and not fight them by attempting to raise a lawn in a hot dry climate, for example. If you are moving to a warmer climate the two main points which you need to consider are that planting times are considerably earlier than you are used to and also that many flowers need protection from the scorching effects of the sun's rays. This can be provided by selecting their area with care in relation to the house, or by planting trees and shrubs in strategic positions.

Soil types will vary enormously even between one side of a plot and another, so it is not possible to generalize. Most plants and flowers are fairly tolerant of differing soil types as long as they are not too extreme and fertilizers can usually make good for any natural lack of nutrients. However, if your soil is rather dry and sandy with a considerable lack of sufficient humus then from a long term view it makes sense to import better topsoil, or improve what you have by digging in compost or peat.

Select your plants and flowers with as much care as you would give to choosing wallpaper for your house, because the latter is the internal decoration and the former the external decoration. Take note of the height of flowers as stated on the packets and graduate your sowings or transplanting from highest at the back of a border to lowest at the front. Consider which colours blend together and which will clash. It is not advisable to have more than one strong scented flower in any one position, as this tends to confuse the senses. There is no necessity to avoid annual flowers, as in a warm climate they will mostly seed themselves if you give them sufficient time.

There is also no reason why you should not plant vegetables if you have the space and the inclination. They often take a day or two to reach the markets and shops even before you buy them and there is further deterioration in freshness if you are not purchasing daily. Admittedly greens such as cauliflower, broccoli and cabbage will not grow in summer in a hot climate, but there are other alternatives at this time such as beetroot, carrots, melons and tomatoes. Vegetables taste so much better when freshly picked from your garden at the time when you are ready to use them. It is rather pointless to use all your ground to grow potatoes, as these are cheap and deteriorate little in transit. Whatever you grow remember that a butt is useful to catch rainwater, as this is better for plants than tap water which has additives and is charged by meter according to usage.

Finally, rather than just planting ornamental trees and shrubs, give due consideration to fruits and nuts, as these can be quite attractive. Your range of choice will naturally be limited depending upon whether your local climate is temperate, sub-tropical or tropical. However, in the popular retirement areas of southern Europe you should have a choice in many places of orange, lemon, fig, cherry, plum, apricot, pomegranate and almond to mention just a few possibilities. In addition, there are a great many countries where you can have grapevines trained up a pillar or a trellis.

21 Pets

In retirement a pet is often a great comfort to a couple and an even more valuable companion to a single person. For those countries where there is a security problem a barking dog, particularly a large breed, can be a deterrent to burglary. For most of the popular retirement areas there are few, if any, restrictions on the importation of domestic pets providing that the correct procedure is followed and quarantine is seldom necessary in continental Europe. However, in fairness to your pet, if you do take it abroad be reasonably certain that you intend to stay, as there is often a long period of quarantine necessary to reimport the animal into your home country such as Britain. As a result, a large number of pets are abandoned abroad because the owners decide that they cannot afford the expense of quarantine. This can be a greater cruelty than such owners complain of in ill-treatment by others.

The documentation necessary varies from country to country and this can be arranged by your veterinary surgeon, who will give or obtain the necessary certificates and have them legalized at the appropriate consulate. It is quite possible that you could drive right across Europe telling the customs officers at each border post that you are importing pets and they would all shrug their shoulders and say 'So what?' Nevertheless, it is better to be in possession of the correct documentation and not rely on such casual attitudes, or quarantine and expense could follow.

If you decide to leave your pet at home, or do not have one, then it is possible that you may obtain one after your arrival abroad. This may be by purchase or perhaps an unwanted young animal. If you are seeking a pet bear in mind that it is very likely there will be an animal sanctuary in your area where abandoned pets, often pedigree animals, are in need of an owner and they may have to be destroyed if they do not find someone to accept them. If you retire to an exotic location you may even rear a young wild animal. When I worked in Uganda for an aid organization during the Karamoja famine my pet was a gecko which spent most of its time on the bedroom wall eating mosquitos and other insects. I find wild creatures very approachable and sometimes before dawn when it was rather cool the gecko would get into bed with me and I would find it there in the morning.

Remember that most domestic pets are capable of bearing cold weather, but some suffer considerable discomfort in high temperatures. This is particularly the case with certain large breeds of dogs with long, thick coats, especially if they are overweight and of advanced years. If your pet comes into this category it is advisable to give careful consideration to whether it would be better to leave it at home with relations or friends.

Finally, if you do not intend to remain in your retirement home throughout the year, before you obtain a pet give some thought to how it will be looked after in your absence. Perhaps you have neighbours who will accept this task, or there may be kennels or a cattery in your area. A villa exchange may be possible with people who will look after your pets. My cat was originally left as a small kitten, unable to fend for itself, by a couple who spend half of the year in their homeland. Remember that domestic animals do not feed themselves and the cost of food for them is not inconsiderable; so is it going to be within your contracted budget? Inevitably there are also likely to be veterinary expenses at times. A young animal is desirable which you can train properly. Strays which have run in a wild pack are best avoided, as they may well continue to be unruly and vicious.

22　Future Problems

You would be very fortunate indeed and the exception rather than the rule if you had no problems whatsoever during the whole of your retirement abroad. Hopefully, any difficulties will be of a minor nature and you will have the assistance of neighbours or friends in helping you to overcome them. There is a saying, 'forewarned is forearmed', and we may be able to be prepared to meet some problems if we know in advance what they are likely to be. So what difficulties is it likely that we may have to face as retired expatriates?

An obvious one is medical problems, as retired people seldom grow old without them. There are a number of ways in which we can prepare. Firstly, we can select a retirement area which is beneficial in relation to any ailments which we possess already. People suffering badly from arthritis, for instance, have often been known to throw away walking sticks and even crutches shortly after moving to a dry, warm climate. It is quite obvious that you should avoid unhealthy countries, as elderly people are often more vulnerable to diseases and infections. Secondly, serious consideration should be given to taking out private medical insurance (even if you are covered for reciprocal state health service benefits), the main reasons being that you will certainly feel more comfortable and receive better individual attention in a private room than in a public ward. Also there are often very long waiting lists for operations in state hospitals. Beware of insurance companies which cut you off from further participation at a certain age. And thirdly, bear in mind that it is very likely that you will need or can benefit from sheltered housing at some stage of your retirement. Consequently, either purchase such property initially or make certain that you plan your finances to be able to buy when the appropriate time arrives.

Bereavement is a problem which just about every couple will face eventually, as we are all mortal. Consequently, it is not a problem which we can avoid, although there are two ways in which we should be prepared. One is that a retired couple should not be completely wrapped up in each other to the extent of cutting themselves off from all other friends and company, or bereavement will be all the more difficult to bear. Another is that you should anticipate any financial problems which may result from bereavement, such as the cost of a funeral or the imposition of inheritance tax. Funerals are almost universally expensive (even for a very simple ceremony) and if the cost is likely to present difficulties then comprehensive funeral insurance can usually be taken out for a modest annual premium. Bear in mind that unlike in Britain most other countries do charge inheritance tax on transfer between spouses at death and the rates are often high, besides commencing at a low level. Be prepared for this eventuality by means of life assurance or making the necessary investments.

Loneliness is often a result of bereavement or divorce, and is much more likely to occur in an isolated location where you have few neighbours who can speak your language. It is also often connected with boredom, which is discussed next, as the more spare time which you have on your hands the more you will feel its effects. For a person living in a community there is little or no excuse for loneliness, as many other people are in the same situation and it is just a question of making the effort to talk to people and being friendly and hospitable towards them. For those who have great difficulty there are usually singles nights or clubs, which are often advertised in the expatriate press. Firm relationships frequently develop from the initial postal contact of penfriends.

As mentioned above, boredom often leads to an escalation in the pangs of loneliness, although a couple who are not lonely can both be bored by lack of sufficient outside interests. Which brings us back to my earlier remarks that it is essential to plan well in advance the activities in which you will engage during retirement and to select an area to live where there are enough interests. Living abroad is completely different from taking a holiday in the same country. During the latter you will want to unwind and relax; as a permanent resident, sunbathing all day soon becomes boring.

Probably one of the most compelling reasons for retiring abroad is the climate in your home country not being to your liking throughout the year. Wherever you move there is likely to be a period during which the local climate is uncomfortable. India and south-east Asia has the sticky monsoon. Spain is very hot in summer and much of Italy experiences quite severe winters. The moral of this is that you should not regard the climate of a country as being continuously as you have experienced it on vacations, because practically everywhere is subject to seasonal variations. The first point to make is that it is important to ensure before purchasing a property that it is capable of being made comfortable in varying climatic conditions without excessive expense. Secondly, if you have an uncomfortable season then consider taking a holiday elsewhere at this time if you have sufficient funds, as a change of scene is likely to do you a lot of good both physically and mentally. For those on a restricted income consider a property exchange vacation, as the only real cost may be that of travel. Home Link International has a subscription of less than £40 and many members in a wide range of countries. Addresses of local agents can be obtained from the author.

Finance will almost certainly become a problem (and a severe one at that) if you ignore the future effects of inflation upon your lifestyle. This matter requires the careful attention of everyone who retires abroad and it is of such major importance that a later chapter of this book is devoted specifically to the matter. What other financial problems are you likely to face? A serious one could arise if you have to change properties for various reasons in the future, such as to move into sheltered housing, necessitating the availability of additional funds. Investments should be made at an early stage so that they can grow in value to provide adequate resources to meet such eventualities.

What aid organizations exist to assist you with various difficulties? The answer depends very much upon the country in which you live. For those people in receipt of a state retirement pension many governments have concluded reciprocal health and social security agreements, which give access to the same facilities which are enjoyed by nationals of your country of residence, although language difficulties can inhibit communication. Often expatriates have formed aid organizations such as HELP. Contact in your area can be obtained from local newspapers, ministers of religion and community offices. If you have spare time on your hands they will almost certainly welcome your assistance and it is much more satisfying to give help than to just receive it without any return. Communities should band together in a organized way to provide mutual assistance during periods such as hospitalization and convalescence on a rota basis, as the burden can often be too severe for just one neighbour or friend to bear. If your committee does not take the lead in this respect then do so yourself, as it is very simple to arrange.

23   Insurances

Personally I am not a believer in insurance funds for investment purposes, as their performance is mostly mediocre to poor. Nevertheless it is commonsense to insure against other risks. Basically what you are doing when taking out insurance is to pass the risk to someone else for a consideration called a premium. The latter is assessed statistically according to past claims and set at a level to provide the insurer with a margin of profit in average circumstances. In certain cases where the risk is not large and you consider that in your case the probability of loss is much less than average then you may decide to be your own insurer, by saving the premium and accepting the level of risk. An example of this is in deciding to take only the compulsory third party vehicle insurance rather than the comprehensive, which carries a high premium inflated by many accidents caused by unskilled and careless drivers in dense traffic conditions to which you may not be subject.

I have no life assurance because I prefer to provide for this eventuality in other ways. It may be appropriate for many other people and it is one way in which provision can be made for liability to inheritance tax. The 'with profits' life assurance offered by British companies has defensive advantages, as a sum is locked in each year and cannot subsequently be lost in a stockmarket plunge. With term life assurance the total premium is lost to the insurance company if the assured does not die within the stipulated time scale. Probably endowment is a better alternative; unless there is a large contingent liability for a limited period, such as on gifts possibly liable to death duties if the donor does not survive for a certain time.

One of my clients does not insure his house, as he considers the risk of fire to be low. However, this is not the only risk and loss of your home is a serious matter for the sake of saving a premium of only 0.2 per cent per annum. House and contents insurance is surely a necessity on overseas property, especially considering the incidence of crime. Do not necessarily assume that foreign insurance companies have the same financial stability as those in your home country as they may not be subject to a similar level of governmental supervision in relation to their risks and reserves. Be especially careful of small insurance companies operating over a very limited area and recommended by developers to all their clients. This means that they have a massive risk concentrated over a small field, which negates the first principle of insurance to spread risk. Also check that you have full cover before you pay any premium. I have seen foreign policies stating 5 per cent cover on damage caused by a burglary, rising to 10 per cent and 25 per cent for other risks; this is merely conning you that you have any proper form of insurance. The Overseas Property Insurance Services Europlan, underwritten at Lloyds of London, for instance, provides comprehensive cover with premiums of £2 per thousand for buildings and £6 per thousand for contents in Spain and Portugal. If you have a swimming pool be careful to ensure that your public liability insurance is adequate, as loss of life is possible in a pool.

As the title of this book is 'Retirement Abroad' I intend to exclude the discussion of health insurance schemes which are available only to working expatriates. The first decision which you will need to make, if you decide to have private medical insurance, is whether to select a local or a more international policy. Some local insurance companies are not very well capitalized and accept large risks for low premiums, resulting in bankruptcy. Often cover is restricted to just one province and extension to the whole country is only possible with advance agreement. Frequently additional charges are made for cover in another country. Claims experience by many people is not good, some being refused with very flimsy excuses. For instance, a friend of mine required hospital treatment for gallstones and although he had no previous record of such problem the local insurance company refused to pay the bill, saying that the gallstones were forming when he joined the scheme.

Brief details of various popular international schemes are tabulated below some of which are open to adults of all ages up to the maxima stated:

Policy	Maximum benefit	Maximum age	Europe 70 years old
BUPA International Senior Lifeline	£100,000	Enrol before 75	£1,125
Europea-IMG New Expatriate Health Care	£500,000	Enrol before 75	£400
Exeter Hospital Aid Society (Basic)	Individual limits apply	Enrol before 75	FR £204 FS £420
ExpaCare Senior International Health Plan	£25,000	No limit	£1,025
International Health Insurance	£200,000	Enrol before 80	£1,102
Medicare International Health Plan (Basic)	£1,000,000	No limit	£1,201
PPP International Health Plan (Basic)	£100,000	No limit	£1,049
Trans-Care International	£150,000	Enrol before 70	£245
WPA (Teak)	£9,000	Enrol before 60	£494

The Exeter is cheapest on the FR scale, but this only provides a maximum of £500 for surgeon's fee and £80 per week for hospital accommodation which is unlikely to be sufficient in most countries. It must be stressed that the above only gives abbreviated features for general comparison purposes and it is essential for you to study the fine detail of the conditions attaching to each policy to ensure that your requirements are covered. For instance, the Exeter scheme does not cover emergency repatriation, but Trans-Care's does. In some cases the premium varies according to age, but with Trans-Care and the Exeter it does not, although the latter charge a once only scaled fee to those joining over the age of 65. The premium may or may not vary according to geographical area, North America often being subject to higher charges. The size of your family is also a relevant factor when considering premiums as many companies charge per person. Trans-Care have a 10 per cent discount for a family group exceeding two persons and Exeter cover dependants for approximately one-third extra.

Funeral insurance is often available on a local basis for a very modest premium considering the high cost of even a basic funeral. One of the most useful aspects of this insurance is that sometimes the company makes all the arrangements, which is a very comforting consideration in a foreign country speaking a different language when the grief of bereavement is enough to bear. Watch to see whether cover is cut off at an advanced age, or premiums escalate extremely sharply at that stage.

Vehicle insurance is discussed on the basis that you are resident abroad for the majority of the year and you drive a car registered locally. In those circumstances the legal position is usually that it is mandatory to effect insurance with a local company. Again the problem often arises of non-payment of claims, or excessive delays only terminated by costly legal action. You may find that some insurance companies from your home country have registered subsidiaries locally and it is quite possible that they will offer you an immediate no claims bonus built up over the years, even with another company. Fully comprehensive insurance may only be available on new cars and it is often expensive. You may therefore weigh this cost against the risk of accepting only third party insurance, particularly if your vehicle is not of high value.

Travel insurance will probably not be of interest to, or necessary for, retired people living permanently abroad in just one country, as their house and contents insurance most likely covers the majority of their risks. It should be borne in mind that travel insurance is, in fact, a composite insurance covering various matters such as flight delays, baggage loss, medical treatment and theft. It is a fairly simple matter to arrange travel insurance with a local travel agency, although it is sensible to consider whether you really need it. For instance, flight delays may not concern you, baggage loss is usually covered by the airline, you may have medical cover abroad and you carry travellers' cheques to minimise the effects of theft. In such circumstances it may be rather pointless to duplicate insurance cover. For those people who make many journeys each year consider a multi-trip policy, as this can produce a considerable saving over individual arrangements.

24   Legal Matters

On the subject of property purchase procedure I do not intend to go into a great deal of detail here, mainly for two reasons. Firstly, laws and practice vary considerably from state to state and it is not helpful to generalize. Considerable detail on the legalities of house purchase is given in Appendix II for the popular retirement countries. And secondly, I do not want you to gain the impression that a 'do-it-yourself' job is in any way satisfactory when buying a property abroad. In the foreword to my first book, *A Villa on the Costa Blanca*, Edward McMillan-Scott, who is the Member of the European Parliament for York and the European Parliament rapporteur on cross-border property purchases, writes:

> The problems of buying a property in Spain, or even renting one, are candidly set out in this book. I have been examining this sector for over two years and I have seen much misery among the expatriate community. Almost always, those who encounter problems have been too trusting.
>
> My conclusion is this: before committing any money to property, take professional advice. In the European Parliament we are working hard with the Spanish authorities to squeeze out bad habits, but they die hard.

Except perhaps in the USA, where there is a very high level of consumer protection, a buyer always needs a solicitor when purchasing a property abroad. Do not listen when a developer or agent tells you that a solicitor is 'not necessary' as this advice is not given in your best interests and could well indicate that they have something to hide, such as plans for a new motorway through the property. Never accept a seller's offer to use his solicitor, because you need a different and independent person to look after your interests. The fact that a notary is used does not negate the need for independent legal advice, as the notary's usual function is to see that the interests of the state and its laws are observed. The exception is in France, where it is usual for a *notaire* to handle the contract on behalf of both buyer and seller, the costs being shared. I do not think that there is any point in instructing your solicitors in your home country because, unless they have a regular link for property purchases in the relevant state, then two professional fees are likely to result rather than just one. If you have difficulty in finding a local solicitor who speaks your language then try your consulate in the area, as they will certainly have a list of possibilities, although they will not make recommendations or a selection.

If you buy property abroad it is advisable to use your foreign solicitor to make a local will covering your possessions in that country, whether or not you have a valid will in your home country. Again do not rely on a 'do-it-yourself' job, as unfamiliarity with the local laws could well cause enormous legal difficulties which prove greater than dying intestate. The main reason for making a local will is administrative convenience as the cost is likely to be quite low, whereas the expenses of legalizing a foreign will are often ten times as much. As many popular retirement countries impose inheritance tax upon surviving spouses it is advisable to incorporate a clause stating that if your spouse dies within thirty days of your death then the estate passes to next of kin.

During a temporary absence certain matters may need to be dealt with and you may consider giving a power of attorney to your solicitor, or other person you trust. It is not advisable to put an excessive amount of temptation before anyone and so the power of attorney should not be a general one authorizing any action in relation to all your possessions, but only a specific one concerning the matter in hand. It is quite usual to empower a solicitor to register deeds on your behalf. Ensure that the registration is going to be in your name and not his, as the Code Napoleon (which is the basis of laws in the Latin countries) does not recognize nominees and the concept of beneficial ownership, the person registered having absolute title. There may well be other urgent matters which could arise during your temporary absence, such as filing tax returns and payment of rates, for instance. If they cannot be dealt with by a simple banker's order then you may need to engage a suitable professional person. In some countries there is a legal requirement to appoint a fiscal representative in your absence. If you are going away for a long spell check the security of your house. Consider arranging regular inspections, particularly if there are narrow time limits for notifying insurance claims. Should you have stated on an insurance proposal form that you intend to live in the property on a permanent basis then tell your insurance company how long you will be away, what security arrangement you have made and confirm that you have unoccupancy cover.

Many people who have sold property or a business retire at an early age, so that a birth in the family of a retired couple is far from an impossibility. If it occurs abroad then the local laws for registration should be followed, which generally involve taking the certificate received from the doctor or midwife to the local town hall, where a birth certificate is usually issued. This should then be taken to the parents' consulate for registration, together with other relevant documents such as both parents' birth certificates and their marriage certificate plus passports. Normally it is possible for baptism to be arranged locally, according to faith.

Neither is marriage unusual for retired people, as quite often it is only at this stage that they find their partner. Remember that common law spouses are frequently not recognized in many Latin countries as having any legal relationship and inheritances passing to them on death are often subject to the highest rates of tax applicable to unrelated people, which can be up to 84 per cent of the value of the property. In some of the Latin countries a church wedding is only possible providing that at least one of the parties is a Roman Catholic. Otherwise it may only be possible for them to be married at a Civil Registry. This can be followed, optionally, by a church ceremony which is not recognized as a marriage. If either party has been divorced then probably a solicitor will be required to deal with the legal complications. Those resident in southern Spain or Portugal may like to know that British or US citizens can marry at a registry in Gibraltar. Your local consulate will supply details of the procedure.

As in any country, if you are contemplating divorce then you should certainly consult a solicitor. Most countries accept the usual grounds, such as cruelty, desertion and adultery. A judgement will normally be given in the local court on such matters as maintenance, shares of common property and the custody of children in the absence of voluntary agreement on these matters. Finally, as always, death – which should be registered at the town hall by someone who knew the deceased, presenting the doctor's certificate giving the cause of death. The local death certificate which is issued should be taken to the deceased person's consulate and a death certificate obtained which is valid in the country of origin. The estate should not be distributed, as this is a matter for a local solicitor. Remember that inheritance tax is often payable by the surviving spouse within strict time limits.

25 Banking

The two main requirements which expatriates have from banks are that they provide the services which are required and they do so at a reasonable cost. A client of mine with £20,000 to invest had never previously had a bank account in his life. Retired expatriates always need at least one bank account in the country in which they live and preferably also another externally, whether it is in their country of origin or in an offshore centre such as the Channel Islands. The latter is absolutely essential if exchange control regulations exist in the country in which they live. Even if this is not the case an offshore bank account is desirable to minimise or eliminate taxation of interest. For instance, a British person permanently resident abroad is still subject to British income tax on all income arising in the UK, which includes England, Wales, Scotland and Northern Ireland, but not the Channel Islands and the Isle of Man. Consequently, it is better to close bank accounts on the mainland and instruct your bank to transfer the balances to their branch on one of the islands.

Consider which types of accounts you require offshore, whether current, deposit, interest-bearing current or high interest cheque account, in order to manage your liquid assets as efficiently as your investments. In case you wish to shop around for a high interest cheque account with the features which suit you then the major conditions are tabulated below:

Bank	Minimum initial deposit	Minimum additional deposit	Minimum cheque	Interest credited
Bank of Scotland, PO Box 588, St Helier	£2,500	£250	£250	Monthly

Bank	Minimum initial deposit	Minimum additional deposit	Minimum cheque	Interest credited
Barclays Bank, PO Box 9, Douglas	£1,000	None	None	Quarterly
Barclays Bank Finance Co. (J), PO Box 191, St Helier	£2,000	£250	£250	Quarterly
Cater Allen Bank (Jersey), PO Box 476, St Helier	£1,000	None	None	Monthly
Guinness Mahon Guernsey, PO Box 188, St Peter Port	£1,000	None	None	Quarterly
Hill Samuel, PO Box 63, St Helier	£2,500	None	£200	Quarterly
Lloyds Bank, PO Box 10, St Helier	£1,000	None	None	Monthly
Midland Bank, PO Box 14, St Helier	£2,000	None	£100	Half-yearly
National Westminster Bank, PO Box 12, Chelmsford	£500	None	£100	Quarterly
Robert Fleming (IoM), 3 Mount Pleasant, Douglas	£2,500	None	None	Monthly
Royal Bank of Scotland, PO Box 678, St Helier	£2,000	None	None	Quarterly
Standard Chartered Bank (CI), PO Box 89, St Helier	£1,000	None	None	Quarterly
TSB Channel Islands, PO Box 597, St Helier	£2,000	None	None	Quarterly
Tyndall Bank (IoM), PO Box 62, Douglas	£1,000	None	None	Quarterly

Bank	£1,000	£5,000	£10,000	£25,000	£50,000	Paid
Bank of Scotland IoM	1.75	9.11	9.11	9.11	9.11	Monthly
Barclays	7.0	7.7	8.4	8.75	8.75	Quarterly
Cater Allen	9.0	9.0	9.0	9.0	9.0	Monthly
Guinness Mahon	8.75	8.75	9.25	9.625	10.0	Quarterly
Hambros, Gibraltar	—	4.0	7.0	7.5	8.0	Quarterly
Hill Samuel	—	9.25	9.25	9.25	9.25	Quarterly
Lloyds	5.0	8.0	9.0	9.25	9.6	Monthly
Midland	—	6.4	7.85	9.06	9.54	Half-yearly
National Westminster	6.125	6.625	6.75	7.25	7.25	Quarterly
Robert Fleming	—	9.0	9.0	9.0	9.0	Monthly
Royal Bank of Scotland	—	7.5	8.25	8.7	9.2	Quarterly
Standard Chartered	6.0	8.0	8.5	8.75	8.875	Quarterly
TSB	—	8.5	8.5	9.0	9.0	Quarterly
Tyndall	9.0	9.0	9.0	9.0	9.0	Quarterly

Some of these banks offer similar facilities at other offshore centres and not only at the address given. US dollar accounts, specifying a minimum of US$ 2,000 upwards, are available from Bank of Scotland, Cater Allen, Robert Fleming, Midland, Standard Chartered and Tyndall. Also Fleming offer Deutschmark and yen accounts; while Midland have a choice of twenty foreign currencies in cheque deposit accounts. You will appreciate that the rate of interest on all accounts will fluctuate with changes in the bank rate and possibly more frequently. High interest cheque accounts are not a suitable medium for long term investments as the rates are not fixed and they fluctuate approximately in parallel with the bank rate. Consequently in a falling interest rate environment, such as must be expected at the present time, your income is constantly shrinking. Purely as an example with a British bank rate of 10.5 per cent the following H.I.C.A. rates are on offer at 27 February 1992: see table opposite.

Regard should be given to the frequency of payment of interest, as this affects the annual return. For instance, Midland may appear to be offering a higher rate on £25,000 than Robert Fleming, but as the latter account credits interest monthly the compound annual rate (CAR) is 9.38 per cent per annum. Another point to bear in mind is that the Isle of Man has a deposit protection scheme with compensation payments, whereas the Channel Islands have none. Another reason why bank accounts and building society deposits are not suitable for investments is that the funds inevitably depreciate in value due to inflation while they are earning interest. For instance, recently when UK inflation was standing at 10.9 per cent per annum the best rate obtainable was 12.5 per cent, so the real return on leaving money in such an account for a year was only 1.6 per cent. If, meanwhile, the exchange rate in your country of residence appreciated against sterling then you could well be in negative territory with an actual loss on the deposit. Your banking pattern and the consequent charges are important; also the position regarding interest if your balance falls below the minimum requirement is very relevant. The Bank of Scotland credits a lower rate and the Midland account earns no interest. With the latter you would be far better off with one of their new interest-bearing current accounts if your balance is likely to hover frequently above and below the H.I.C.A. minimum. Most of the British High Street banks now offer a complete expatriate package. This is 'lazy man's investing' if you accept it, as the bank will almost certainly invest all your available money only in its own restricted range of funds, which frequently do not perform as well as other funds, both in regard to yield and capital appreciation. Unfortunately, they have the bank's interests mainly in mind and you do not receive unbiased and independent advice regarding the many hundreds of funds on which a consultant can advise.

We now turn our attention to banking in the country of residence, the main banks being listed under state headings in Appendix II. The most important consideration is communication. It is no use having the best bank in the country if you cannot discuss your affairs with the staff due to a language barrier. So ensure that more than one senior member speaks a language which you understand. Discussions with other expatriates will assist you to find a local bank which is efficient, has reasonable charges and does not delay your transfers for an excessive time. Various accounts are likely to be available and these are given in more detail for the popular retirement countries in Appendix II. Care should be taken in selecting the correct type of account in states with exchange control regulations in force, such as Portugal, otherwise your funds could be locked into a blocked account, or you may be breaking the law. Often it is not advisable to hold large sums in a local bank far in excess of anticipated needs, as withholding tax (which can be as high as 25 per cent) is frequently deducted from interest. If the country does operate exchange control then it is certainly not advisable to bring in all your funds, as you will be limited in the amount which you can take out on trips abroad.

Transfers of funds from one country to another can be quite expensive in relation to the sum involved. For this reason it is sensible to investigate the alternatives available to employ the most economic method. Regarding the payment of British state retirement pensions abroad, the Department of Social Security in Newcastle has recently concluded arrangements to pay pensions in certain countries free of bank charges and you should certainly take advantage of this scheme. If your British bank has a local branch, transfers are often cheaper and quicker than going through foreign correspondent banks. Another economic method is by means of the Giro Bank system for payment by the local postal authorities. Some foreign banks accept your personal cheque drawn on another country, although your account is not necessarily credited immediately and a cheque usually takes about three weeks to clear. If you arrange a telegraphic transfer from your home country the cost on a relatively modest sum is likely to be about £15; a mail transfer being slower and slightly cheaper.

Credit cards are not used as much as in the USA and UK in other countries, although their acceptance is now spreading rapidly through northern Europe. As far as southern Europe is concerned it is the rare exception rather than the rule for retailers to take them in payment. Some large department stores and hypermarkets issue their own credit cards for in-house purchases, as do certain banks for wider acceptance in such places as filling stations. The internationally-recognized credit cards can be useful for obtaining cash from many banks.

Eurocheques find general acceptance throughout northern Europe, although again their use in the southern half of the continent may be mainly to obtain cash to the equivalent value of £140 or so at banks. The use of Autocheque Cards to obtain cash up to the stated limit is being extended to cash machines abroad, particularly as a result of links forged between banking groups in various countries.

26 Exchange Control

Exchange control regulations are gradually being dismantled throughout the European Community, as this is an eventual condition of membership. However, do not necessarily expect them all to disappear within the EC by the end of 1992, as Portugal has recently been granted an extension of controls until 1995. Outside of the European Community some relaxation has occurred recently in countries such as Sweden, although in other parts of the world exchange control could well remain for a very long period.

What are exchange control regulations? These are rules made by certain countries and supported by the force of law to prevent or to restrict the movement of money in all its forms into and out of the country and to control foreign exchange transactions. If you visit Algeria you have to complete a declaration stating not only your cash and travellers' cheques, but also your jewellery and even your wedding ring. Little do the authorities know that on their southern border the Tauregs smuggle camel loads of gold across the Sahara desert, which is impossible to police.

When you are purchasing property in a country where exchange control regulations are in force it is essential to follow the correct procedure for importing funds for this purpose. The rules vary from state to state and are subject to frequent change, so it is important to obtain up-to-date advice on this matter from your local solicitor. Generally speaking it is usual for the funds to be placed in a particular type of account and your local bank provides a certificate of importation, which is sometimes incorporated into the deeds of your property. Failure to follow the correct procedure and to obtain the relevant bank certificate could well lead to problems if you later sell the house. Remember it is the buyer who is likely to have the difficulties, so if the seller asks for payment in a currency other than the local one consider what possible difficulties could arise for you later if you agree to this request. It may well be that the seller is avoiding capital gains tax by this method. In Spain, as from 1st January 1991, a purchaser of a house from a non-resident individual or company with no permanent establishment in Spain is now required to withhold 10 per cent of the purchase price against possible tax liability of the seller. Remember that when you obtain a residence permit in a country subject to exchange control rules you are probably only allowed to operate a non-convertible bank account locally and you would be breaking the law to do otherwise, or to retain foreign currency accounts within that country.

Repatriation of money to another country, such as surplus funds or the proceeds of a property sale, is only allowed under exchange control regulations providing that the relevant rules have been strictly observed. If this is not the case then you could very likely discover that the money is in a blocked account, which prevents you from moving it out of the country either permanently or for a very long period. Therefore it is important that you give careful attention to this matter when purchasing a property, bearing in mind that unexpected circumstances may arise which necessitates an unplanned sale of the house, or much earlier than originally anticipated.

As stated in the previous chapter, it is advisable to have a bank account outside the country and not bring in the whole of your funds. There are two main reasons for this. Firstly, it leaves you with money available to invest anywhere in the world to the best advantage, whereas local investment may produce poor returns and be subject to withholding tax on dividends or interest up to 25 per cent. Secondly, you then have adequate funds available for vacations and trips outside the country, however long their duration. There is a holiday allowance under the exchange control rules, which is probably adequate for a short trip, but it may not provide you with sufficient money for travelling a longer distance or for an extended period.

Again there is no point in mentioning here the current sums which you are allowed to take out of various countries, as the regulations are subject to constant changes. Your local bank will have up-to-date details and it is advisable to consult them when you are planning a trip and arranging the finance. A Spanish businessman tells me that he takes a suitcase full of money out of his country at frequent intervals. No matter what he does, the actions of the Tauregs, or the workings of the 'rucksack economies' of Central America, you should not exceed the allowances in the exchange control regulations, whether travelling by air, sea or land to another country. Point one: it is dangerous to carry large sums in cash, with the risk of theft. Point two: the whole of your funds will be confiscated if discovered and random body searches are likely in the effort to combat drug trafficking. Point three: the law prescribes heavy additional penalties in the form of fines and/or imprisonment for breaking exchange control regulations.

27 Inflation

Inflation is likely to be the most serious matter to affect the lives of the vast majority of retired expatriates and I am not exaggerating the position in any way when I say that the problem at its worst could well be a matter of life and death, because you cannot afford to buy sufficient to eat. Consequently, you should read this chapter with the utmost care and then make your plans to cope with inflation in the future. Do not say, 'It may not happen'. Inflation is taking place today as you are reading and it will go on happening in the future; the only matter in doubt being the actual rate of it.

The most frightening aspect of inflation is its insidious nature and the stealthy way in which it creeps up on you almost unnoticed. A rise of a few pesetas, escudos, lire or francs on this item, then on that and before you realize it just about everything has increased in price. As a retired expatriate living in another country a few points must be borne in mind regarding the local inflation rate. It must be appreciated that this is a figure which is politically highly sensitive, as it is often used in fixing wage demands, rent increases and for many other purposes throughout the economy. As a result it is in the interests of the government to manipulate a low rate by imposing controls on certain items used in the index. However, the latter is based on the spending pattern of local nationals, which is likely to be very different from the budgets of expatriates. The latter are also charged higher prices than nationals for identical items in many places. Furthermore, you may well be living in a popular vacation area where prices shoot up enormously every summer and later fail to return to their former level. So the moral of the above is to regard the official inflation rate with a pinch of salt, as expatriate inflation is likely to be considerably higher.

But just as an example of the seriousness of inflation to our lives, let us take the official inflation rate of a popular retirement country such as Portugal, where it is at present 12.1 per cent per annum and assume for the purposes of illustration that it remains at this level in the future and does not increase. Also we assume that we continue to buy exactly the same things and do not change our spending pattern.

Year	Income	Expenditure
1993	£10,000	£10,000
1994	£10,000	£11,210
1995	£10,000	£12,566
1996	£10,000	£14,086
1997	£10,000	£15,790

You see from the above just how quickly your costs increase by well over a half. Perhaps by 1997 you can find an extra income of £5,790 a year in order to cope. But what if our total maximum income is only £10,000 per annum and we were spending it all on living costs in 1993? Economise, did you say? All very well in theory, until you get down to specifics. Then you find that you have already been careful in your spending and not wasteful. You have to pay your rates promptly or there will be a surcharge. You cannot reduce your expenditure on electricity, gas and water. So what are you going to cut down on – food? How are you going to produce an overall saving of almost 58 per cent in your total expenditure by 1997 – eat about a quarter of the quantity which you did in 1993? That is what I mean by inflation being a matter of life or death.

For a person in receipt of a British state retirement pension it is true that the amount is uplifted annually by the rate of UK inflation. Stress must be placed on the final words of the latter sentence. If the local rate of inflation in your country of residence is higher then you will have to fund the differential. UK inflation was just over 4 per cent in early 1992 and officially projected to fall. This is welcome for those who remain there, but it is not good news for British expatriates retired in other countries such as Spain where inflation (officially, even though Spaniards laugh at the underestimate) is nearly 7 per cent and rising. As a result annual increases in British state retirement pensions in the future are likely to be well below the increased cost of living in many popular retirement countries. British people retiring to such countries as Australia, Canada, New Zealand, Norway or South Africa should remember that their state pension will be frozen at the figure originally granted and not increased. This would soon make it practically worthless with even modest and average inflation levels in those states.

Historical rates of inflation in your country of residence are of interest to a certain extent, as states tend to suffer a consistently high or low level. In general, socialist governments tend to produce higher inflation than more right wing ones. I am not preaching politics here, but merely stating an economic fact. Any reference librarian will be able to produce books for you which chart inflation rates over the years for most countries.

Current inflation rates are given weekly in *The Economist* newspaper, but only for the dozen or so largest economies in the world; which include France, Italy and Spain, but not Portugal or Greece. The embassy and consulates will be able to tell you the up-to-date figure, or you can return to the reference library for information. Inflation rates available at the time of writing are given in Appendix II.

However, you will well appreciate that our main concern is with likely future trends, rather than with past or current inflation rates. This is a terribly complex matter to forecast, even by an economist, because it results from the interaction of a great many diverse factors. Taking just one, I should say to people retiring to the states of southern Europe to expect high inflation, because of their total dependence on imported oil which affects transport costs and hence all goods. The most an average person can do is to err on the side of caution and assume a future inflation rate higher than the current one. It would be a serious mistake to underestimate the ravages of inflation upon your lifestyle. It is pointless to take any notice of official forecasts for inflation because, apart from the fact that this is a politically sensitive matter, an honest admission of future high inflation is self-defeating. For instance, when the Brazilian government frankly tells its citizens that it expects inflation to increase to 80 per cent per annum then you know it is very likely that the actual figure will exceed 250 per cent. The reason is that traders anticipate high inflation and discount it by raising their prices at an early stage. Inflation is self-multiplying, not just by arithmetical progression but by geometrical progression and the whole process snowballs like a runaway express train.

People who are in receipt of a fixed income as their sole means of support are the ones who will be most seriously affected by inflation. They will continually have to make economies, until the point is reached where this is no longer possible. Then they will have to sell their property and move into a cheaper one. This may give respite for a time, although a worse scenario is that they will have to return to their country of origin and depend upon national assistance. There is some hope for them if they act at an early stage when their income exceeds their expenditure and they invest the surplus. Building society and bank deposits are not suitable for this purpose, because they merely produce additional income (which is no more than a temporary stopgap), whereas the capital gain is nil on these accounts and it is such gain that is required to combat inflation on a continuous basis. As stated already, the return of 12.5 per cent per annum gross on such accounts at a time when UK inflation is 10.9 per cent gives a real return of only 1.6 per cent a year. After taxation the return is negative.

So, providing that you are not in the unfortunate position of having only a fixed income which just provides for your present needs, what should your strategy be? Firstly, itemise your present income from all sources, such as state retirement pension, occupational pension, bank and building society deposits, investments, etc. Secondly, make estimates of your likely income in future years. Assume the uplift of state pension to be no more than 3.5 per cent in future years. In regard to company and occupational pensions, although they are often termed 'inflation proof' an independent survey recently found that they increased on average by considerably less than half of the current UK inflation rate, and so it would be unwise to expect a larger increase in the future. As far as building societies and bank deposits are concerned, the British bank rate is expected to fall from 15 per cent in October 1990 to 6 per cent by the end of 1993. Because all money market rates work in parallel you should expect the top rate obtainable on a high interest account to fall from 13 per cent to 4 per cent in just over three years. As a result you could well find that your total income next year is likely to be considerably lower than at present. This comes as a shock when you raise the cost of your expenditure by a factor of at least the current rate of inflation.

That is why it is absolutely essential to plan your finances well in advance and not wait for an intolerable situation to arise. If you delay until the bank rate falls then you miss the capital gain which results at that time on British government securities ('gilts') or on bonds. For a long dated security you can probably reckon on a substantial capital gain for every one per cent when the bank rate falls. In addition, you are locked into the higher yield obtained at the time when you invested.

When you have made the above projections for future years on the basis of the best information available you are then in a position to consider what your correct investment decisions should be. If you discover that you need additional income immediately then you should invest the appropriate sum in gilts or bonds. Offshore gilt funds produce a yield of up to 17.8 per cent per annum at present (although do not expect such high rates to be available for much longer), or various bond funds have yields between 4 per cent and 11.4 per cent per annum. An example is as follows:

Current expenditure		£10,000 p.a.
Less income:		
State Pension	£3,000	
Occupational Pension	£5,000 =	£8,000
Shortfall		£2,000 p.a.

Current yield on a high income gilt fund is 17.8 per cent. Therefore calculation is £2,000 × 100 ÷ 17.8 = £11,236 being required for investment in gilts to secure this additional income. Round up to £12,000 to cover unexpected items.

Any additional capital available should be invested in offshore equity funds for growth. It is true that stockmarkets fluctuate from time to time, but you should be able to look forward to an average annual return of at least 22 per cent taking a long term view over a period of about seven years. If you are concerned about risk then various funds are available which guarantee the return of at least 100 per cent of capital invested, and even some which guarantee the highest value reached by the fund during its lifetime. Invariably obtain independent advice regarding investments and it should cost you nothing. No such decisions should be made without giving consideration to their currency of denomination, for the reasons given in the chapter which follows concerning fluctuating exchange rates.

28 Exchange Rates

A Swedish person permanently resident in Sweden receives his salary in krona and all his expenditure is in that currency. Similarly, a British man living all the time in the UK is paid in pounds sterling and that is what he spends for shopping and other costs. Neither of them probably worry unduly about how their domestic currency fluctuates in value against other currencies. It is extremely important to remember that when you retire abroad you enter an international situation. Your income probably arises in your country of origin and when you transfer sums to your state of residence the funds are converted at the ruling rate of exchange into the local currency, which you need to pay your bills. Consequently, fluctuating exchange rates are of the utmost importance to retired expatriates and it is therefore advisable to know how they work.

To take an oversimplified model by way of illustration (because rates fluctuate due to the interaction of a complex collection of factors, including the level of productivity in different sections of the economy, inflation rates, the level of money supply, national budget surpluses and deficits, interest rate differentials, capital flows and gold reserves) we will consider a country with a booming manufacturing output. This production sells well abroad, because the low value of the state's currency makes the goods competitive and when these goods are paid for large sums of other currencies flow into the country, which far exceed the state's foreign payments. Hence a substantial balance of payments surplus builds up and it becomes a 'strong' currency, which many foreigners wish to hold rather than their own weaker currencies. And so additional money flows into the country above the level generated by the trade surplus, which pushes up the exchange rate to a high level. Because of this change the goods now become expensive abroad, sales fall, a trade deficit opens and the balance of payments becomes adverse; its currency changes to a weak one in consequence and the exchange rate falls. Then the cycle repeats itself. In fact it is rather more complicated than that, because politicians tinker with the economy and do such things as raise interest rates to attract international capital, or lower them to deter foreign investment.

The result of all this is that currency fluctuations can be (and often are) violent and extreme. British people in recent times have seen the value of sterling depreciate against the Spanish peseta by 16 per cent in one year; when inflation of over 7 per cent is added their purchasing power has diminished by nearly a quarter in just twelve months, which is a very serious matter. Some currencies have exchange rates which are firmly fixed or loosely linked to another strong currency. For example, certain Far Eastern states peg their currencies against the US dollar. Some Scandinavian countries 'shadow' the Deutschmark and the Swiss franc is part of the 'Deutschmark bloc' of currencies, although Switzerland is not part of the European Community. This does not mean that such currencies are insulated from fluctuations, merely that they experience the movements of the strong currency to which they are pegged. Other currencies float freely.

An extremely important point to bear in mind is that not all currencies can fall in value at the same time, as they are self-balancing. If one falls then this is compensated in the system by another rising. Sterling is likely to rejoin the Exchange Rate Mechanism of the European Monetary System and readers may be wondering how this is likely to affect its future performance. That does not rule out fluctuations, because both sterling and the peseta can vary by up to 6 per cent either way against the mean; the limits for other currencies in the system being $2\frac{1}{4}$ per cent. Consequently the British and Spanish currencies can diverge by up to 12 per cent. Unfortunately this is not the bottom line on possible currency exposure risk, because currencies can still be devalued when they reach the limits. What joining the E.R.M. does do for sterling is to impose a political discipline in regard to inflation (although it must be said that the present Conservative government has taken a very considerable time to control inflation considering that this is the professed major aim of its economic policy) and to deter industries from conceding inflationary wage demands which were previously accommodated by a depreciating currency. Curiously, I think that the major effect on sterling's entry in the E.R.M. will be upon the US dollar and the yen. The five major currencies used for trade and investment are dollars, yen, pounds, Deutschmarks and Swiss francs. Three of the 'big five' are now in the same bloc, which will give them international stability. As previously stated, all these currencies are self-balancing which leaves the remaining two to take the full brunt of fluctuations. Think of these five currencies as a see-saw, three of which form the solid concrete base which anchors it to the ground, the other two being the extremeties of the plank which can swing through a wide arc.

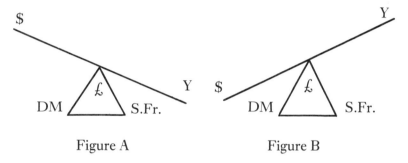

Figure A   Figure B

In both diagrams the Deutschmark, pound and Swiss franc are all boxed in within narrow limits. In figure A, when the dollar is high the yen falls correspondingly low. Conversely, in figure B at times of a weak dollar there will be a very strong yen.

Knowing all the above, what do retired expatriates do to protect themselves from the currency exposure risk implicit in moving abroad? Whether they realize it or not, they will adopt one of three possible strategies: either passive, defensive or aggressive. A passive approach is probably adopted by the vast majority of retired expatriates, mostly through resistance to change and ignorance of the currency risk to which they are exposing themselves. What is the result? Their fortunes, or just as likely misfortunes, are tied inevitably to the one currency in which all their incomes and investments are denominated. They will suffer all the traumatic battering to which their one currency is subjected by speculators in the international currency markets. Every time this currency plunges their standard of living will fall dramatically. As a retired expatriate the main thing you want is peace of mind. The last thing you need is to be kept awake at night worrying that when you go to your local bank the next day you are likely to look at the board listing foreign exchange rates and find your currency has fallen so low that when you change your pension cheque it does not produce sufficient local currency to pay your bills. This is the danger for the 'one currency expatriate'.

In contrast, a defensive (or neutral) stance involves having your deposits and investments denominated in various currencies to roughly equal proportions. The purpose of this is not necessarily to make a currency gain, but to prevent an overall currency loss, bearing in mind that if one falls in value then another must rise. I consider the absolute minimum for this purpose to be three currencies; US dollar, yen and one of those in the European Monetary System. Much better stability would be obtained from a range of five to ten currencies. This arrangement will assist you not only in regard to capital protection, but also in connection with revenue funding. If you go to the bank and discover that sterling is weak, with a low exchange rate, then you can change dollars or another currency and keep sterling in reserve until it improves. The important point is that you have a choice: which you do not have with a passive approach.

An aggressive (or positive) stance is the most advanced stage and this involves making conscious and ongoing decisions regarding the probable future strengths and weaknesses of various currencies, to weight your portfolio with a mix of currencies in different proportions. It would not be unfair to label this approach as a form of currency speculation, but it produces the best results if you correctly forecast future movements. The problem for average persons is that they do not have sufficient experience of the workings of the international currency markets to be right more than about half of the time. When they are wrong it could involve a currency loss. Consequently, this approach should only be adopted with the advice and assistance of an independent financial consultant who is knowledgeable not only regarding investments, but also concerning currency markets.

In any case, currency decisions should be linked to investment decisions and neither should be considered in isolation – the reason being that the overall return is the gain or loss on the investment, plus the currency gain, or minus the currency loss. For instance, a loss of 2 per cent on the yen is acceptable if a Japanese fund produces a gain of 48 per cent. Conversely, a low yield of 3 per cent on a Swiss bond may be necessary to obtain a gain of 20 per cent on the Swiss franc. This matter will not be enlarged upon further here, as it is more relevant to a succeeding chapter on investments. Generally speaking, larger gains will be made from the latter than from currencies. Nevertheless, currency gains can be very substantial and rapid. The optimum is to make the right investment decisions denominated in the most beneficial currencies.

It would be an omission to close this subject without giving the most dire warning that you should not take out a foreign currency mortgage for a property purchase without financial advice, which is completely independent of that given by the mortgage company. Some of the latter do give cautions, although few stress adequately the extremely serious nature of the considerable currency risk exposure you are undertaking, which is open-ended and unlimited in its possible extent. At first glance it may seem like a good idea for an English person to take out a mortgage expressed in Swiss francs because the rate is only 9 per cent. However, strong currencies have low rates and weak ones have high rates, so that the cost of buying appreciating francs to service the mortgage can far outweigh any savings on interest differential. Ideally, you should take out a mortgage denominated in the currency in which the majority of your income arises.

29 Taxation

Before proceeding to consider investments we should firstly bear in mind our taxation situation; because most people pay taxes unless they are fortunate to live in a place, such as Andorra, which is a tax haven. The important point to bear in mind is that just because you leave your country of origin you do not automatically and with immediate effect escape taxes in that country. Even if you comply strictly with all the rules, it often takes a high proportion of retired people at least three years before they are officially classed as not resident for tax purposes. If one of your main reasons for moving abroad is to reduce your taxation, then you should firstly ensure that taxes are not likely to be more onerous in your new country of residence than in that of your origin.

As far as British taxation of its expatriates is concerned, the Inspector of Taxes is fully entitled to (and usually does) wait three complete tax years after retired persons have moved abroad before regarding them as non-resident for UK taxation purposes. The action which such people should take when they are aware of their date of leaving Britain is to obtain from their local Inspector of Taxes form P.85 and complete this, as it starts the process moving and also acts as a claim for any overpayment of tax. During the interim three fiscal years you should be extremely careful not to contravene the rules for escaping residence and ordinary residence mentioned below. Having done that and eventually achieving the desired status, your overseas earnings will be exempt from taxation in Britain. However, most income arising in the UK will still be subject to British tax. The main exemptions are on certain British government stocks. Remember that the Channel Islands and Isle of Man are not part of the UK for tax purposes, as they have their own fiscal authorities which are quite independent. This is why offshore investment in these and other locations becomes extremely useful. It is certainly to the advantage of most British people to transfer their assets out of the UK and there is no need to move them to their country of residence, as an offshore centre is ideal for this purpose. The timing of taking capital gains requires very careful planning when moving abroad, unless the liability is extinguished by exemptions and allowances. The main exemptions are your principal private residence, possessions sold for less than £6,000 and disposals of UK government securities. There is an annual tax-free allowance of £5,800 per person after indexation relief for inflation. In addition, there may be business retirement relief, or previous losses, to offset. If a balance remains which is subject to tax, then certainly attempt to delay taking the capital gain until you achieve non-ordinarily resident status, because it will then exempt you from such UK tax. If there is a possibility that you may wish to sell a business as a going concern at some time in the future before moving abroad and there is likely to be a Capital Gains Tax liability, then you should obtain professional advice regarding the incorporation of the business at the earliest opportunity, so that it does not appear to be an artificial transaction merely to avoid tax.

Although not many people are aware of the fact, the UK is a very attractive tax haven for non-British people living there, providing that strict attention is given to the rules for avoiding tax. If such a person came to the UK with the intention of staying for more than three years they would be regarded as resident and ordinarily resident from the date of arrival, income before and after that date being apportioned in the British fiscal year, but a full year's personal allowance being granted. Providing such a person retains a non-UK domicile (which is usual, as you will see from the explanation which follows) they would be taxed on both income and capital gains remitted to the UK, but not on capital so remitted. Consequently, their best tax planning arrangements would be to transfer as large a sum as possible to the UK in advance of their arrival to purchase a property if they so wish, plus funds to cover expenses and living costs for the maximum period. They should open three separate bank accounts and make absolutely certain that these are not tainted in their purity by mixing funds from different classes. One should receive income and this should not be remitted to the UK or it will be taxable. The second should be a receptacle for capital gains, which again should not be remitted on pain of tax. The final account is kept for pure capital, or funds redeemed at cost, or on which there has been a capital loss and any of this money can be remitted to the UK without suffering British taxation.

Many people think that just because they go to live abroad they will cease to pay all further taxes, but this is not the case unless they have a very low income or move to a tax haven. In the past some states were the latter by default or omission, because they often failed to collect taxes even from many of their own nationals. This is now changing completely as a result of advances in technology and the computerization of fiscal records. If you are resident abroad your global income is likely to be taxed and this will include income which may be exempted from tax in your home country, such as interest on British National Savings Certificates. Similarly, interest which is paid gross, as on deposits with banks and building societies, will be chargeable to tax. Almost invariably there are deductions and allowances available which you must claim, as they may not be given automatically. It is almost always beneficial to employ a local tax consultant, as this can save much more than his or her fee, particularly if you are not very familiar with the local language and the fiscal laws. For instance, in Spain a deduction of around 15 per cent of the cost of buying a property is available, although few people realize this.

We now need to define the terms domicile, residence and ordinary residence as used for taxation purposes, as these are different from the usual understanding of the words in everyday speech. Domicile is important because it decides your liability for British inheritance tax. The fiscal definition of domicile is not just the place where you live, but it is more akin to the state which you regard as your 'home' country. However, your view on this may well differ from that of the tax inspector, who will not be prepared to state an opinion during your lifetime on a hypothetical liability to inheritance tax, but only to make a decision on your death in connection with an actual assessment. It is a very complex matter and one on which you should take expert professional advice if a substantial estate is involved. Putting it very simply, domicile is not necessarily fixed for the whole of your lifetime, as it may change from a domicile of origin to one of dependence or one of choice at various times. The domicile of origin which you acquire at birth is normally the same as that of your father, which is not necessarily the same as either his or your residence, nationality or passport at that time. A domicile of dependence may be acquired by a child or by a woman married before 1 January 1974. A child under sixteen takes any new domicile of the parents on a provisional basis. When the child reaches sixteen this becomes a domicile of choice, unless steps are taken to re-establish the domicile of origin, or a different domicile of choice. A domicile of choice is by far the most difficult to attain, because you must produce incontestable proof to the Inland Revenue that you have severed all your links with your country of origin. This does not necessarily preclude an occasional short visit, although the retention of even one club membership would be enough to refute a change of domicile. There is no point in a British person attempting to change his or her domicile if the global assets of the estate are less than £150,000, because bequests of up to that sum are free of British inheritance tax. In many other countries even small amounts are taxed, rates can rise to as high as 84 per cent and transfers between spouses are liable to inheritance tax.

Residence is usually defined for taxation purposes as where you live for more than six months of the fiscal year. The latter runs from 6 April to the following 5 April in the UK, although it is often the same as a calendar year commencing on 1 January in many other states. Strictly speaking, if you spend 183 days or more in the UK in a fiscal year then you are regarded as being resident for the whole of that year, although by concession the British Inland Revenue normally divides the tax year into periods of residence and non-residence when you move abroad. Even if you spend less than 183 days in the UK in a fiscal year, you may still be liable for British tax if you make what are termed 'substantial and habitual' visits or have accommodation 'available for your use' in the UK, however short the visit, even if for only one day. Visits are regarded as 'substantial and habitual' if they average ninety days a year over four consecutive years. So you can spend a maximum of 182 days in the UK in one year, as long as you counterbalance this with short visits in other years. Accommodation 'available for your use' is defined as being a permanent arrangement, whether or not you actually use the rooms. It would probably not infringe this stipulation if you stay with members of your family, rent accommodation on a short term basis, or retain property as long as it is let for a fixed period with no right of possession on your part.

Ordinary residence is very closely linked to the factor of continuity. Consequently, the UK Inland Revenue interpret it as being the same as habitual residence. This body normally insists on a waiting period of at least three complete tax years before regarding a retired expatriate as being non-ordinarily resident. As long as the rules regarding visits and accommodation are not contravened the status will be applied retrospectively to the date of leaving the UK and any tax overpaid as a result will be refunded. However, as very substantial sums could accumulate over such a long period, it is preferable to transfer assets which produce income or capital gain to an offshore location at the earliest opportunity. This is particularly important remembering that even after you achieve non-resident and non-ordinarily resident status, income arising in the UK will still be subject to British tax.

Most countries of the world, with a few exceptions, charge some form of tax upon income. Details for the UK and for some of the popular retirement countries are given in Appendix II. Some states have rates which are quite progressive to a high level and so it is important to consider in advance of moving whether you will be paying more income tax than in your country of origin. Those with an extremely high income may well decide to live in a tax haven such as Andorra, which has no impositions upon income.

Your country of residence may or may not levy a tax upon capital gains, or possibly it will add such accretions to income for the purposes of assessment. Normally such rises in value only crystallize for the purpose of capital gains tax when the asset is eventually sold, although a market value of shares and stock may be taken for wealth tax purposes. Check whether your intended state of residence gives an indexation allowance, because if it does not then you will be paying tax upon inflation. Some countries charge capital gains only on property sales and not on the disposal of securities and other assets.

Wealth tax is not so common throughout the world as either of the above impositions. It may possibly be levied upon both residents and non-resident property owners, perhaps under different rules with separate allowances and at varying rates. Take care when filing a wealth tax return to give the official value of your property if this is the basis of assessment, as this could well be considerably less than the current market value or the price which you paid for it.

Inheritance tax often amounts to a great deal more in a foreign country than in your home state. It is important to estimate your potential liability and to make any necessary provisions for paying this tax upon your death, otherwise your surviving spouse may be left with no alternative other than to sell the property in order to pay the inheritance tax due. Remember that you can reduce the assessment by half if you register the property jointly in the names of both spouses at the time of purchase. Alternatively, at this early stage you may decide to put the property in the name of your children, so deferring any charge until one of them dies.

Withholding tax needs careful consideration, although strictly speaking it is not a separate tax, but an obligatory deduction on account of possible tax due. As one example, in Spain a deduction of 25 per cent is made from bank deposit interest before it is paid to you. The problem is that you may not be due to pay any income tax, because of a low income or the deduction of allowances. In some countries it is not possible to reclaim the tax in such circumstances, or it is only received after excessive delays. The solution is simple – invest in such states as the Channel Islands or Luxembourg where there is no withholding tax.

Value added tax (under various names) has spread rapidly throughout the world, particularly because imposition of this tax is a condition for entry into the European Community. It may well be levied at vastly differing rates on various classes of items, such as whether they are considered to be essentials, ordinary items or luxuries (the latter sometimes including cars). In some countries certain classes of goods, such as food-stuffs, may be exempted or zero rated.

Rates have disappeared in the UK, being replaced by a poll tax called the Community Charge, although the latter will be subject to future change. If you retain a property in Britain, although you retire abroad for part of each year, give careful consideration to the length of time which you spend in the two countries if you wish to escape this charge. In many other countries a contribution towards the cost of public services is required under a form of rating system, often based upon the official value of the property. Where an incomplete development has not yet been adopted by the local authority then such matters may be dealt with by a committee of owners and a community charge levied.

The system and sequence under which calculations are made can be much more important than just the nominal rates of tax. As an example, the minimum rates of income tax in both the UK and Spain may previously have appeared to be the same at 25 per cent, but as allowances are given against gross income in Britain and against tax due in Spain the tax payable on identical incomes can be considerably less in the latter country.

If you are tax resident in one country and paying taxes in another remember that it is very likely you can offset tax paid in the latter against tax due in the former state, providing that the two have signed a double taxation treaty. For instance, Britain has concluded double taxation treaties with:

Antigua	Gambia	Malta
Australia	Ghana	Mauritius
Austria	Greece	Montserrat
Bangladesh	Grenada	Namibia
Barbados	Guernsey	Netherlands
Belgium	Hungary	New Zealand
Belize	India	Nigeria
Botswana	Indonesia	Norway
Brunei	Irish Republic	Pakistan
Bulgaria	Isle of Man	Philippines
Burma (now	Israel	Poland
Myanmar)	Italy	Portugal
Canada	Ivory Coast	Rumania
China	Jamaica	St Kitts
Cyprus	Japan	Sierra Leone
Denmark	Jersey	Singapore
Egypt	Kenya	Solomon Islands
Falkland Islands	Kiribati	South Africa
Faroe Islands	Lesotho	South Korea
Fiji	Luxembourg	Spain
Finland	Malawi	Sri Lanka
France	Malaysia	Sudan

Swaziland	Tunisia	USSR
Sweden	Turkey	West Germany
Switzerland	Tuvalu	Yugoslavia
Thailand	Uganda	Zambia
Trinidad &	USA	Zimbabwe
Tobago		

Such a treaty may permit the payment of pensions, interest, dividends or royalties as a gross amount, or subject to a lower rate of tax. So a British person resident abroad should obtain the necessary form from the Inspector of Foreign Dividends, Lynwood Road, Thames Ditton, Surrey and have it stamped by the local tax office abroad, possibly only after obtaining a residence permit. Remember that they will be checking later to confirm that you have declared this gross sum on your foreign tax return.

30 Investments

Unless you have very large pensions, which are able to cope with the ravages of inflation throughout the whole of your lifetime, then you are going to need investments to help support you at some stage during your retirement abroad. Where those investments are located is of vital importance to their net return and that is why we have just studied the taxation implication in such detail. The investments may be in your country of origin, in which case a currency fluctuation risk will be involved, as the investments will be denominated in a different currency from the one in which your expenditure is expressed. Consequently, if your home currency weakens in value against that of your country of residence then this can adversely affect your standard of living, such as happened recently with the 16 per cent depreciation of sterling against the peseta in one year. What investments are likely to be available in your home country? Obviously I cannot give a comprehensive list for every state in the world, so let us just take Britain as an example, which is probably typical in its range. Building society and bank deposits can be used for a small sum which it is necessary to keep liquid for emergencies, when cash may be required in less than about ten days. Neither of these types of deposit is suitable for coping with the long term effects of inflation, as you can only draw out the capital which you put in, depreciated as it inevitably is by inflation. As clearly shown in Chapter 27, with a previous rate of 12.5 per cent per annum gross on a high interest cheque account and UK inflation running at 10.9 per cent, the real gross yield is only 1.6 per cent per year. Even if paid gross the interest will be subject to tax in your country of residence, so that the real net yield will be less than zero, it will be negative. In other words you will be losing money by making such deposits. Some people say, 'But I must do this for reasons of security'. Banks and building societies are not necessarily secure, as they can easily go into liquidation or bankruptcy. All four large UK High Street banks have loaned billions of pounds to Third World states and it is extremely doubtful whether they will even receive the interest, much less the return of capital sums. They are also highly exposed to a drop in the property market and in 1975 one of the 'big four' was in considerable danger of going under for this reason. Similarly, property represents a very high proportion of the assets of building societies and in the recent situation of rising unemployment, interest rates and inflation, plus falling house prices, they are finding that a sharply increasing number of borrowers cannot pay their mortgage instalments and often a larger sum has been advanced than the current market price of the property, even in the unlikely event that it could be sold. Many hundreds of 'thrifts' (the equivalent in the USA of building societies) have recently become bankrupt in a falling property market and the deficiency is expected to exceed 160 billion dollars. British National Savings are secure, but the returns are often poor and in some cases recently well below the current inflation rate, so again you are losing money by making such investments, particularly as they are taxable abroad. UK government stocks ('gilts') have a yield a little above or below the inflation rate. The problem may come later when your stock reaches the maturity date and there is no suitable alternative to replace it. An offshore gilt fund is preferable, as it has a portfolio of various stocks maturing in different years which are managed to provide continuity of high income. Finally, there are unit trusts and investment trusts which on average do not perform quite so well as offshore funds and suffer from the twin disadvantages of being denominated only in sterling (so presenting a currency risk) and also being subject to UK taxation.

You may decide to make some investments in your country of residence. In this case there will be no currency loss if all your expenditure takes place there. Conversely, the disadvantage is that there will be no currency gain, even against a currency such as the Portuguese escudo which is weak against almost every major currency in the world. The local economy may be a poor or slow moving one and in this case it is an unnecessary restriction to confine yourself to investments in such an environment, when all the dynamic world is open to you. A major drawback to investing in the country in which you live is that withholding taxes may mean that you have to pay the tax at an exceptionally early stage. You may say, 'Well, I would have to pay it anyway!' but time is money and by delaying the payment of tax for a year or more you can earn very substantial returns. To give an example; say you are an expatriate living in Spain and you have the equivalent of £100,000 which you place on deposit with a Spanish bank earning 12 per cent interest payable annually on 31 March and subject to a withholding tax of 25 per cent. Therefore, on that date the bank deducts £100,000 × 12 ÷ 100 × 25 ÷ 100 = £3,000. Now if you had an identical investment abroad on which the interest is paid gross you would account for this to the Spanish Inland Revenue on 31 May of the following year. Consequently, you could invest this £3,000 in an offshore gilt fund for fourteen months with a yield of 17.88 per cent per annum, so producing £3,000 × 17.88 ÷ 100 × 14 ÷ 12 = £625.80, which you would not otherwise have had.

The third alternative of investing offshore is by far the best for expatriates. Not only does it open up the whole world to you, but also your investments can be denominated in any of the major currencies, so managing your exchange rate risks. In addition, redemption proceeds on almost all funds are obtainable in about ten days, and all payments of interest, dividends and capital are made gross without any tax deductions. If you are concerned about possible risk then guaranteed funds are available. However, a check on the performance of over one thousand of the main offshore funds shows that in only five cases in the seven years ended on 1 May 1992 was the return below the par investment level, three of those being commodity funds and another a property fund. With less than 1 per cent risk of partial loss, diversification can protect you, because the substantial gains on the remaining 99 per cent far more than offset any small depreciation in value of a few. How do the returns compare? Let the facts and figures speak for themselves. In the case of banks, building societies and National Savings these are the current UK figures. As far as the offshore funds are concerned the dividends are the current figures and the total returns are the average per annum over the past seven years to eliminate temporary fluctuations.

RETURNS ON INVESTMENTS – MAY 1992

Investment	Interest/ Dividend % p.a.	Capital appreciation % p.a.	Total return % p.a.
British banks			
Deposit	2.5	Nil	2.5
High Interest	6.1	Nil	6.1
Building Societies			
Ordinary	8.5	Nil	8.5
Three months notice	9.6	Nil	9.6
National Savings			
Ordinary	5.0	Nil	5.0
Investment	8.5	Nil	8.5
Bonds	10.2	Nil	10.2
Certificates	8.0	Nil	8.0
Offshore Funds			
Gilt-edged	8.8	5.4	14.2
International bonds	6.7	10.4	17.1
International managed	2.9	9.2	12.1
International equity	1.5	20.1	21.6
UK equity	3.0	12.2	15.2
North American	1.0	17.1	18.1
Australian	2.5	3.9	6.4
Japan	1.1	18.2	19.3
Far Eastern	1.0	36.1	37.1
Hong Kong	2.4	44.0	46.4
European	1.0	26.9	27.9
Commodity	1.8	4.5	6.3
Managed currency	6.5	9.6	16.1
Sterling currency	9.9	5.4	15.3
US $ currency	3.3	4.1	7.4

As can be seen, the fixed interest funds (gilts and bonds) have done quite well considering that this was a period of rising interest rates, which is the worst time for them. Almost all the equity funds (except Australia) have produced enormous returns on a consistent basis. Commodities have disappointed largely due to gold's poor performance and are mostly best avoided. The currency funds have more than matched the best alternatives available in those respective currencies.

A little more detail is now required concerning the various classes of offshore funds. Gilts are British government stocks and experts will tell you that there is no safer kind of security in the world. Gilts are best for income, because they currently produce yields of up to 17.8 per cent per annum. They are far from the ideal vehicle for protecting yourself against inflation, as the average capital appreciation is often not greatly above inflation level. As with all funds the timing of your investment is crucial and the ideal period for purchasing gilts is when interest rates have reached their peak and are falling, or better still about to fall. Then you can probably expect a capital gain every time the bank rate falls, in addition to the income. Conversely, it is an unsuitable time to invest in gilts when interest rates are low and rising.

Why should you invest some of your funds in international bonds when the yield is lower than on gilts? Firstly, because the capital gain is usually much higher, with the result that the overall return is considerably above that for gilts. Secondly, to diversify the currencies in your portfolio to protect the value of your income and capital, as gilts are only available in sterling. Bonds evidence a loan to a sovereign state, supranational body or to a corporation on which interest is payable. Consequently, there is greater continuity of income than from dividends of a variable nature on equity funds.

Growth funds are mainly investments, that is, they consist of shares in commercial companies. Unlike a bond, which is evidence of a debt, a share confirms that the registered holder is the owner of a part of the assets and income of the company. Of course, there are risks in investing in just one or a few companies; so an offshore equity fund, like a similar unit trust fund ('mutual fund' in North America), buys shares in about thirty to fifty different companies to obtain an average return for that particular market. The figures given in the above table are also averages and some equity funds have produced spectacular returns of up to 925 per cent over the last seven years. In my own portfolio I have recently taken gains of 97 per cent over two years and 72 per cent over one year, such profits not being unusual. Again timing is important, as a typical economic cycle lasts for seven years, with five good ones and two poor years. So invest as a boom starts and sell to move into bonds or currency funds when a recession threatens. Do not wait until a sudden crash.

International managed funds often consist of various

proportions of all classes, including gilts, bonds, equity, commodities and currency funds, the percentages in the total holding being varied constantly by the fund manager in the light of current market conditions. The performance depends upon how well the manager carries out this function. They are a good risk-spreading ploy for unsophisticated investors with limited funds available after securing the necessary income.

Umbrella funds are popular with 'do it yourself' investors who wish to construct their own managed portfolios, because the 'super fund' has various classes of sub-funds between which you can switch as desired at little or no cost. Actually, there are dealing costs which the static investor ultimately pays. You are gambling if you are an amateur and lack professional advice on switches. And remember that it is not like putting a few bob on a horse – it is your future with which you are gambling.

Most currency funds produce better returns than banks, because the former aggregate numerous investments of £1,000 or more so that they can obtain the much higher interest rates available on the money market for large sums. With this type of fund do not expect very much capital gain or loss. It is useful for an interim period when switching between equity and bonds at times unsuitable for an immediate change. Such funds are also ideal for contracted property purchase, possibly by instalments, when the liability is expressed in a foreign currency, as they protect you from unfavourable exchange rate movements. A few currency funds deal in forwards and options; these have produced enormous returns of up to 230 per cent in one year recently. Of course, the risks are much greater with this type of fund, although tranches with a minimum 100 per cent return of capital guaranteed are available at times.

I cannot stress too strongly that fully independent financial advice is essential before making any investment. You are not likely to find it from your bank manager, because he is under an obligation to push the bank's own limited range of funds, even though their performance is poor in relation to both income and capital appreciation. Neither will you obtain it from the so-called 'consultants' employed by fund managers, as they are just salesmen for only these funds. Even in Britain where there is a self-regulation system, any fool can register as a financial consultant and this is no guarantee of their qualifications, experience or competence. They are also permitted to represent just one fund manager. Abroad there are even more 'cowboy' operators. So how do you find a good, competent, independent financial consultant? You can discover whether he is truly independent if he is able to offer you a choice of hundreds of funds, rather than just the range of ten or twenty which one fund manager has available. Competence is indicated by a relevant professional qualification, such as Chartered Secretary or Chartered Accountant, which are to be preferred to an insurance qualification, as insurance funds do not perform very well. Whether he is any good or not you can find out from your enquiries of local people, as a resident permanent member of the community is far more use to you than a 'fly-by-night' who rents a hotel room for occasional consultations. How much will independent financial advice cost you? Probably nothing; as the adviser acts in a similar way to an insurance broker and receives commission from the funds which you select. If you invested directly you would pay exactly the same amount to the fund managers. Very often a financial adviser will supply free information on such matters as taxation.

What is the correct way to go about constructing a portfolio? The first and most important point to make is that everyone is an individual with different needs and objectives, so that there is no 'ready made' portfolio suitable for all. To give proper advice a consultant needs from you full and frank information on such matters as nationality, country of residence, property ownership, overseas visits, tax situation, domicile, age, marital status, children, dependents, occupation, income, pensions and whether index-linked, planned retirement age if not already reached, insurance policies, mortgages, bank accounts, present investments (if any) and deposits, income requirements, liquidity requirements, growth requirements, attitude to volatility and planned inheritance provisions. Working with the above details, the initial step is to produce sufficient income to meet the current budget if pensions and other income need to be supplemented. This is best achieved by a mix of gilts and bonds, for diversification of currencies. Any funds then remaining should be invested for growth. If the balance available is quite small, then it may be necessary to restrict further investments to international managed funds, using a minimum of two denominated in different currencies. Hopefully, a larger sum is left which can be divided to spread investments around the world in the various capital markets, such as North America, Japan, the UK, Continental Europe, the Far East and Pacific area, not forgetting the imprecation in Chapter 28 to select funds denominated in various currencies.

Dividends from gilts and bonds which you need to supplement your income will obviously be drawn. In the case of equity dividends, which are likely to be much smaller as the main objective is capital growth, you normally have a choice regarding payment. It is sensible to have these accumulated in the form of additional shares or units, rather than have the bother of paying various small sums into your bank accounts. If one of your objectives in investing offshore is confidentiality then you should have offshore bank accounts set up to receive these dividends. Accounts both in your country of residence and in that of origin are likely to be open to inspection by the fiscal authorities, often sharing and passing information between themselves. This is not the case as far as offshore bank accounts are concerned.

You will appreciate that there is only a limited amount of information which I can give in just one chapter on the absolutely vital subject of investments, which are your life support for the future.

31   Returning Home

The vast majority of retired expatriates enjoy their life abroad. Unfortunately, a small minority find that they must return to their homeland at some stage. The reasons can include such causes as boredom, loneliness, death of a spouse, missing the company of children and grandchildren, illness of parents or other relations, inflation-induced problems of meeting living costs, or ill health.

Assuming that not merely a temporary return is necessary, it is probable that you will sell your overseas property. Whether you do so for payment in the local, your home state's, or a third country's currency may depend upon your preference, or the buyer's flexibility on this matter. Remember that almost any hard currency is freely transferable into any currency you desire. Unless you have a particular reason for wanting the furniture and furnishings for use in another country, it is normally advisable to attempt to sell the property fully furnished if at all possible. Quite apart from the fact that they are unlikely to be suitable for use abroad, there is the very important consideration of the high cost of removal.

It is highly unlikely that you will want to leave the proceeds of the property sale in that country and the probability is that you will desire to repatriate the funds to your home country or transfer them elsewhere, such as to an offshore centre. If no exchange control regulations are in force for your former state of residence then most likely no obstacle will exist to doing just that; although some countries which demand an exit visa on leaving require confirmation that your local taxes have been paid as a prerequisite for issue. Even if there is exchange control the chances are that you will be able to repatriate the proceeds providing that you have the usual proof of importation of funds to purchase the property in the first instance and you otherwise comply with the regulations. This may well also apply to any capital gain which you have made on the sale; but see below regarding its taxation. If you cannot repatriate the proceeds immediately then it is advisable to consult your local bankers, as they are likely to be the ones who need to seek the necessary permissions on your behalf. Some people overcome the problem by selling to an overseas buyer for a foreign currency to be paid abroad, although Spain has introduced a withholding tax which the buyer must deduct before paying the purchase price.

It may be that you have to return to your homeland urgently as the result of a sudden emergency, so accepting whatever taxation consequences inevitably follow this decision. Alternatively, the necessity may arise gradually over an extended period and in the latter case you could find it possible to decide upon the optimum dates to mitigate your tax liabilities. Again, I cannot give details for every nationality, but just as an example of what is possible with careful tax planning let us take the case of a returning British expatriate. The fiscal law is slightly complicated, although it is worthwhile giving the matter careful attention as large savings can be made. Apart from the three circumstances mentioned in Chapter 29, such a person would be considered UK tax resident from the date of return if he or she returns intending to remain there permanently or for a number of years. Not only UK income becomes taxable, but also global income and capital gains. The extremely important point to bear in mind is that overseas income is taxable under Schedule D, either Case IV or V, both being assessed on the basis of income arising in the previous year. By concession the Inland Revenue restrict the charge proportionally according to the amount of time which the person is resident during the fiscal year. As a result, it is beneficial to arrange your return as close as possible before 5 April, if you have flexibility. Even so, you must expect to receive an immediate tax assessment on overseas income received during the previous year. What can you do to avoid this unexpected shock? The loophole is that, although the normal basis of assessment is on the previous year's income, where there is a new source of income then this is assessed on a current year basis. This gives scope for beneficial tax planning. Investments can be sold before return, possibly 'bed and breakfasted' by repurchasing the identical ones the next day, or preferably by buying new and different investments. In the case of a deposit account, the action which should be taken is to close the account completely, transfer the funds very temporarily to a current account and then open a new deposit account. To give you the flexibility to do the latter without penalty it is advisable to move out of fixed term deposits if the likelihood of return to the UK is a possibility. It cannot be stressed too strongly that UK bank accounts and building society deposits are affected extremely adversely in the case of returning expatriates. There is no concessionary apportionment and a full year's charge is made. Furthermore, it has little or no effect if you close the accounts before returning to the UK. Consequently, it is advisable to close UK deposits when you move abroad and locate them offshore. Alternatively, you need to close them in the fiscal year before that of your return to escape this very unwelcome tax charge, which is completely avoidable with proper planning.

As far as capital gains tax is concerned the ideal objective is to realize gains before returning to the UK (possibly 'bed and breakfasting') and to hold capital losses. Bear in mind that if you have been non-resident for tax purposes for a continuous period of less than thirty-six months then disposals in the fiscal year of your return will be taxable, whether made before or after arrival in the UK. Consequently, if you are affected by this provision it is advisable to sell investments on which there is a gain not later than 5 April in the fiscal year prior to that of your return.

Finally, I trust that you will find you have no need of this ultimate chapter, as the contents of this book are directed mainly towards expatriates who have completely retired.

Author's Note

No one person can be an expert on all subjects. As Confucius said, 'When you reach the stage where you think that you know everything, then you realise that you know nothing.' However, my specialization is finance and if I can answer any of your questions on this subject then I shall be glad to do so if you care to write to me at the address given below.

My sincere wish is that you will thoroughly enjoy your retirement abroad and find this book helpful in some way.

Robert H.V. Cooke F.C.I.S.

770 Rosa
Avenida de Europa 62
Urb. La Marina
E03177 San Fulgencio
(Alicante)
SPAIN

Appendix I

Emigration Checklist

Moving abroad is probably one of the most complicated operations in which you will engage in the whole of your lifetime. Of course there are many variables depending upon principally the country you are moving from and the country to which you are going, besides a host of other personal considerations. However, as a general guide I have set out below some of the matters which will require the attention of British persons retiring to an overseas location. The symbol zero (0) denotes the date of moving abroad. Negative figures signify the number of days before leaving your home country and positive figures refer to days after arrival in the new state.

Earliest date	Latest date	Action	Date initiated	Date completed
−730	−365	Visit various countries which are prospects for retirement and obtain information on such states		
−730	−365	Incorporate your business if it will be sold as a going concern		
−730	−270	Commence seeking a property abroad		
−730	−270	Start learning the foreign language		
−730	−270	Buy foreign dictionary		
−365	−180	Put your property up for sale		
−365	−180	Read library books on country of intended retirement		
−300	−180	Visit property exhibitions		

Earliest date	Latest date	Action	Date initiated	Date completed
−270	−90	Book inspection flight		
−270	−30	Buy a stock of cotton clothing if going to a warm climate		
−270	−30	Make a will in your home country		
−270	−30	Consult a foreign solicitor		
−270	−30	Pay deposit on foreign property		
−270	+7	Open a foreign bank account		
−180	−90	Obtain a five or ten year passport		
−180	−60	Arrange a school for your children		
−180	−30	Arrange payment of an occupational pension into a bank account		
−180	+30	Commence a corre-spondence course, if desired		
−120	−90	Give notice of withdrawal of National Savings Bonds (three months) and Premium Bonds		
−90	−45	Ask DSS about your pension contributions if below retirement age		
−90	−45	Arrange for DSS to pay your pension abroad free of charges		
−90	−30	Arrange documentation to import domestic pets, or find them a new owner		
−90	−30	Renew driving licence, if necessary		
−90	−7	Purchase shortwave radio, if desired		
−90	+7	Buy a local map of your region abroad		
−90	+30	Buy and read a travel guide to the region		
−60	−30	Purchase reading mater-ial, paperbacks, etc.		
−60	−30	Obtain several passport photographs		

Earliest date	Latest date	Action	Date initiated	Date completed
−60	−30	Obtain quotations for storage and transportation of effects		
−60	−30	Open bank account(s) in the Channel Islands or Isle of Man		
−60	−21	Obtain tinted glasses if moving to bright conditions		
−60	−14	Close building society and UK (not Channel Islands) bank accounts		
−60	−14	Obtain quotations for removal in country of origin		
−60	−2	Book flight		
−60	+120	Apply for company or self-employed pension to be paid gross of tax		
−45	−21	Obtain visa application form		
−30	−14	Sell your furniture		
−30	−14	Arrange monthly transfer to a foreign bank, if necessary		
−30	−14	Obtain prescription medicines		
−30	−14	Inform your local Inspector of Taxes that you are emigrating and complete form P85		
−30	−12	Arrange for the disconnection of your telephone		
−30	−10	Obtain Eurolicence or International Driving Permit		
−30	−10	Arrange for your electricity and gas meters to be read		
−30	−7	Arrange storage of effects and keep detailed list		
−30	−7	Arrange payment of storage charges		
−30	−7	Arrange car hire abroad		
−30	−7	Obtain visa, if required		

Earliest date	Latest date	Action	Date initiated	Date completed
−30	−7	Obtain a supply of Euro-cheques, travellers' cheques and foreign currency		
−30	−2	Place subscriptions for magazines, if desired		
−30	+2	Arrange house and contents insurance		
−30	+3	Buy furniture abroad		
−30	+150	Arrange transportation of effects		
−14	−7	Buy good quality tea to carry		
−14	−5	Buy some British stamps so that friends returning can post your letters in the UK		
−7	−1	Cancel your order for milk and newspapers		
0	0	Obtain entrance stamp in your passport		
0	+3	Pay in funds to your foreign bank account		
0	+90	Complete purchase of property		
0	+90	Pay water and electricity connection plus community charges		
0	+90	Arrange gas contract, if desired		
0	+90	Arrange health insurance (optional for pensioners)		
0	+90	Pensioners register with foreign Health Service		
0	+90	Obtain photocopies of your passport, house contract and any other documents necessary for a residence permit application		
0	+90	Apply for a residence permit		
0	+180	Obtain title deeds and registration of foreign money importation for property purchase, if necessary		

Earliest date	Latest date	Action	Date initiated	Date completed
0	+?	Continue paying voluntary pension contributions until age sixty (if not working) or sixty-five, if desired		
+1	+30	Evaluate cars for purchase		
+7	+14	Contact financial adviser and purchase offshore gilts, bonds and/or equities		
+7	+21	Register with consul and obtain certificate of good conduct, if required		
+7	+60	Join sports and other clubs		
+7	+60	Plan your garden		
+7	+90	Obtain quotations for removal from foreign firms		
+7	+90	Obtain confirmation of means from foreign bank, if necessary		
+7	+90	Arrange funeral insurance, if desired		
+7	+90	Consider life assurance and arrange, if desired		
+7	+90	Make a foreign will		
+14	+60	Purchase car, arrange insurance and registration		
+14	+120	Consider satellite or cable television		
+14	+365	Obtain foreign driving licence		
+14	+365	Apply for a telephone to be installed, if desired		
+21	+120	Obtain top soil and start planting your garden		
+60	+150	Collect residence permit, if ready		
+75	+90	Obtain extension of visa if you have not applied for a residence permit		
+300	+645	Complete foreign tax returns		
+365	+730	Apply for second residence permit, if necessary		

Appendix II
Country Information

FRANCE

Climate North of the river Loire there is a typical northern European climate, the exceptions being Brittany and part of Normandy which are milder but very wet. Around the popular retirement areas of Dordogne and Lot there are long warm summers, although winter is foggy and wet. Further south in Gascony they also have wet winters, but warm summers. South of the Massif Central long hot summers and short wet winters are typical except when the mistral, a fierce cold gap wind, blows down the Rhone valley. The Midi region, which includes all of the Côte d'Azur, part of Provence and Rousillon-Languedoc, is almost continuously hot and dry except for heavy early spring rains, winters mostly being reasonably warm.

Languages French. If you intend to live in France it is almost essential to learn this language.

Travel Bureaux *Syndicat d'Initiative* in most French towns.

Business hours 0830-noon, 1400-1930.

Inflation 3.1 per cent.

Local banks Lloyds Bank International (France) plc, International Westminster Bank plc, Barclays Bank S.A., Midland Bank France S.A. and many French banks.

Precautions & problems In France the French people expect to speak only French and they are not keen to use other languages even if they know them.

House purchase procedure If at all possible you should avoid using a real estate agent in your home country, or you may end up paying two amounts of commission. The usual procedure in France when buying a completed property is to obtain details from a local estate agent. The

145

latter will draw up a contract (*compromis de vente*) if the property and its price are to your liking. Before signing this, or any other document, you really should consult a legal or financial adviser. This may be a professionally qualified fellow countryman who has settled in France, or a similar French person who speaks your language and can explain the legal technicalities. The standard *compromis de vente* is binding on both buyer and seller, although regional variants of the standard may not be so. The document will almost certainly give the seller's notary as the person to prepare the conveyance (*acte de vente*), but you should not agree to this. Insist on inserting the name of your own notary so that the two do the work jointly. This will probably not cost you any more, as the two share the fee. Ensure that the contract contains a full description of the property, as well as a plan. The buyer must state in the contract whether or not he is purchasing with the assistance of a loan or mortgage. The contract is automatically cancelled and the deposit becomes returnable if such aid is unobtainable within one month of the date of the contract, this period being extendable by the seller. Deposits are usually fixed at around 10 per cent of the purchase price and the ideal arrangement is to arrange for this sum to be placed in a blocked deposit account for which your bank supplies a letter to the seller stating that, irrevocably, it will pass over the deposit at the correct time. If your bank or the seller will not agree to this arrangement then you should pay the deposit to your notary or the seller's notary, but never to the estate agent or the seller. Study the sale agreement to discover whether the deposit is called a *dédit*, in which case the purchaser may withdraw from the arrangement but will forfeit the deposit. The vendor may also refuse to proceed, although double the amount of the original deposit must be paid to the purchaser in this case. If the deposit is referred to as an *acompte* it is a binding agreement from which neither may withdraw. Take careful note of the contract terms regarding payment of commission, the general rule being that this is for the seller's account unless stated otherwise in the contract. Regional variations whereby the commission is shared or paid by the buyer are common in certain parts of the north, as well as in country areas of the west and south-west. If you are purchasing a property where an element of shared ownership is involved then the *règlement de copropriété* should be supplied with the contract and you are also entitled to ask for a copy of the latest account of service charges. You are unlikely to be kept informed of progress towards completion unless you have your own adviser. It is not necessary to attend the completion in person and you are entitled to appoint an attorney to sign on your behalf; although if you rely on the seller's notary the name on the document is likely to be one of his employees and so nobody is looking after your interests. At completion all the necessary funds, including the deposit and the balance of purchase price, plus a further sum of about 10 per cent of the total to cover notarial fees, stamp duties and other disbursements, must be available. Because of delays in transit from abroad it is advisable to place this sum on deposit with a bank in France earning interest until it is required.

When you buy a property which is not yet complete the above procedure generally applies, although you have additional protection in law as follows. In this case the document is called a *contract de réservation*, although it is a binding contract on which you will lose your deposit if you do not complete, rather than merely a reservation. The maximum deposit permitted is 5 per cent for completion within a year, or 2 per cent if up to two years will be taken, no deposit being allowed for longer periods. Deposits are returnable in certain circumstances, such as the non-supply of any proposed services, the developer failing to sign the conveyance to you by the contract date, escalation in the final price exceeding 5 per cent, or a decrease in area or quality of workmanship which will reduce the value of the property by more than 10 per cent. The price must be stated as firm or subject to variation, the latter only being permitted to the extent of an official index. Stage payments must be specified, giving their dates and maximum amounts, normally payable on the issue of architect's certificates. Outline specifications for materials and equipment must be given, as well as a detailed description of the property. The builder must state what insurance is in force or guarantees available to protect your payments in the event of failure on his part. There are a number of additional points to bear in mind. As payment will extend over a period there is a currency risk involved if you are paying in francs. To cover this you should invest in an offshore currency fund denominated in francs, or place the total purchase price on deposit with a bank in France. As only a very small proportion of properties are completed on time, if lateness will involve costs for you then in a buyers' market you should attempt to insert a penalty clause in the contract. A draft conveyance is normally sent to you one month before completion and you should pass this document to your local adviser immediately to give time for the necessary checks. When the building work is complete you pay the final instalment less a 5 per cent retention. At this stage you have the opportunity to inspect the property to point out defects for rectification and it is very desirable that you should do this in the company of an independent surveyor or builder, so that the necessary work is done immediately and you do not have to wait years for their correction. An average figure for legal costs and fees is about 10 per cent, but it may be much less for certain new property and it could be a fair amount more for other buildings.

Local mortgages   Firstly a stern warning must be given that if you take out a local mortgage and your income arises abroad then you are exposing yourself to a long term currency risk, which is completely open-ended in extent. This is a very serious matter that you should not undertake without proper and skilled independent financial advice, quite apart from any which is given by the lender. On the surface it may seem like a good idea to accept a mortgage on which the interest rate is lower than in your own country; but, in fact, the currency risk far outweighs any small differential. You will have to make your own mortgage arrangements in France, as this is not a service provided by the estate agent or notary. There are no building societies and so local banks are the usual source of loans. Subject to status, a maximum of 75 per cent of valuation may be available on a permanent home, or up to 60 per cent on a property for vacations. Do not rely on a survey by the lender to highlight defects, as this is unlikely to take place. Two types of mortgages are available; either monthly repayments which include interest and part of the capital borrowed, or less frequent interest only payments until the capital amount becomes repayable as a lump sum. Both normally run for about ten to fifteen years. Life assurance cover is mandatory. If you are resident in the UK at present the French bank Credit Agricole arranges mortgages in both francs and sterling through its UK office at 14, St Paul's Churchyard, London EC4 8BD. French law provides considerable protection for borrowers, including a minimum ten day consideration period before acceptance and an offer period of at least thirty days and a maximum of four months. Penalties for early repayment may not exceed official maxima and relief may be available in altered circumstances, including a variation in interest rate within specified limits.

Planning permission & building Obtaining planning permission is a matter for a local professional and almost beyond the capabilities of a foreigner, particularly if the latter is not fluent in French. Nevertheless, foreigners should have at least an outline knowledge of the procedure in order to protect their interests. Planning is now supervised at a local level and almost every authority has a declared planning scheme. The only exceptions are some small communes and here building permission will be extremely difficult to obtain. When you buy land or any property in France a *certificat d'urbanisme* is obtained, which gives density regulations and planning rules. Before building may commence it is essential to obtain *permis de construire*, having careful regard to the strict formalities involved. Within two months of making an application, which gives an opportunity for public objections, a decision has to be given on whether it is granted, refused or deferred. Strictly speaking, delay beyond this time limit implies tacit approval, although this can be overturned within the following two months. The grant is valid for building to commence within a maximum of two years, although it lapses if construction is suspended for over one year. When construction is complete a *certificat de conformité* should be obtained, which officially confirms that the terms of the *permis de construire* have been carried out. The above rules apply in large part to dilapidated properties which need to be restored or rebuilt. There are four main methods of building a property in France. Firstly, you can make your own arrangements with builders, carpenters and other tradesmen. Whether or not you engage an architect this method is not recommended, even if you have professional knowledge, as you are unlikely to be familiar with local working practices. Secondly, if you own land with the necessary permission for construction then you can contract with a builder for the construction of a property. In this case there is a certain amount of protection from the law regarding guarantees for completion and the option to pay by instalments in line with progress on building. Thirdly, you can select an architect to oversee construction. The architect should be of your choice and not the builder's nomination. In addition, legal advice on the contract is essential. Finally, there is the method described above of buying a plot from a developer upon which a property will be built for you.

Utilities, costs and maintenance   Water is drinkable in all areas, although it is hard in the majority of regions. In the countryside the supply frequently comes from wells and you should establish your entitlement before purchasing a property. Mains supplies of water are metered and usually charged for at six-monthly intervals. The cost at around 4½ francs per cubic metre is quite high.

Electricité de France is the monopoly supplier of electricity at 220 volts. Connections are possible in all regions, although the charge for supply is higher in very rural areas. Charges are made bi-monthly, alternate bills being estimated. Reckon on a cost of at least 50 centimes per kWh. Night storage heaters can be run for around 30 centimes per kWh. In addition there is a standing charge. It is advisable to arrange payment by direct debit to avoid any unexpected disconnection.

In some town properties mains gas is available, the charging system being similar to that for electricity. Bottled gas is widely used in the countryside and it is probably much more economical than electricity. Supplies are continuously available, although it is always advisable to have a spare cylinder.

Country areas may well not have mains drainage. Septic tanks are widely used and it is advisable to know where this is located and the facilities for emptying it.

If there is a waiting list for the installation of a telephone in rural areas, priority can be obtained for medical reasons. Elsewhere delays in connection are not normally long. Charges are made every two months and payment by direct debit is recommended to avoid disconnection.

Costs, in addition to standing charges on the utilities mentioned above, include community or service charges if there is an element of shared ownership, property tax and local taxes. Insurance cover is available underwritten by Lloyds of London for a premium of £2.50 per £1000 on buildings and £6 per £1000 on contents, the policy being in English. If you deal with a French company, or with the locally registered subsidiary of a foreign group then the policy will be written in French. The level of maintenance costs tends to be in line with local building costs. In areas of fire risk keep the grass and undergrowth cut short and the land clean or you will receive a very large bill from the State Forestry Department for this work.

Common property Apartments obviously have parts of the building which are in the common ownership of all proprietors, although this concept can also apply to detached, semi-detached and terraced properties which have shared roads, leisure areas and sporting facilities, for example. In these cases the whole is deemed to be a *copropriété* and its organization is regulated by a law which has been in force for twenty-five years with minor amendments. Each *copropriété* has its own rules within the framework of the law (which are set out in a *règlement de copropriété*) and you should obtain and study this document before purchasing a property. The last service charge account should also be available on request.

Administration is organized in a democratic way, with an Annual General Meeting to elect the committee, approve the budget and deal with any other matters. Proceedings take place in French. Powers are often given which you may well feel to be an infringement of your individual rights in relation to your property. Your share of the service charges is normally fixed when the property is built and the sum due is often collected by instalments. You are entitled to appoint a proxy to attend meetings (even if you are in residence) and it may be advisable to do this to protect your interests if you are not fluent in French.

Taxes French income tax rates range from a minimum of 5 per cent on annual taxable income between 18,140 and 18, 960 francs up to a maximum of 56.8 per cent on taxable income exceeding 246,770 francs a year. However, before tax is levied 10 per cent relief is given on state and occupational pensions up to a maximum of about 29,000 francs. Such pensions also qualify for a further deduction of 20 per cent of the net sum after the 10·per cent relief. Pensions received from government departments are taxed differently. A married man is also entitled to relief up to 16,000 francs against French dividends and certain other investment income. New foreign arrivals file an income tax return in February and pay the amount due in September. In subsequent years payment is either by the standard system of one-third of the prior year's tax liability on 15th February and 15th May with the balance payable by 15th September; or, alternatively, by 10 monthly instalments of 10 per cent of the prior year's figure with the balance settled in November and December.

On the sale of a French property at a profit a permanent resident who is moving to another property in France need not be concerned with capital gains tax on the profit, as there is an exemption in respect of your principal private residence in such circumstances. However, the rate of this tax is 33⅓ per cent for non-residents, so if you are moving to another country then your status is of the utmost importance.

As was explained in Chapter 29 it is extremely difficult to change your domicile and this probably only comes about if you show every intention of never returning to your country of origin. Therefore, assuming that you are not domiciled in France, inheritance tax would only be levied on your assets situated in France. With a French domicile it would be assessed on your global assets. Remember that there is no exemption for the surviving spouse. It is assessed upon the individual beneficiaries and not upon the estate. The rate depends upon the relationship of the beneficiary to the deceased. In the case of spouse, child or parent the lowest rate of 5 per cent applies to assets valued below 50,000 francs, rising by stages to the highest rate of 40 per cent on assets over 11,200,000 francs. Most will fall into the 20 per cent band where property is involved. Brothers and sisters pay 35 per cent on amounts up to 150,000 francs and 45 per cent on the excess. It is 55 per cent for more distant relatives and 60 per cent for unrelated beneficiaries. The close relations in the first group are allowed 275,000 francs free of tax. Brothers and sisters are given an exemption on the first 100,000 francs, providing that they have lived with the deceased for a minimum of five years before death happened. All beneficiaries have an exemption on the initial 10,000 francs.

Wealth tax is payable if your global assets exceed 4 million francs and you are a resident. For non-residents to be liable their assets situated in France would need to exceed this figure.

Taxe foncière is a small property tax levied upon the owners, whether or not they are resident. Liability is established on the first day of January and there is exemption for two years after the completion of a new property.

Taxe d'habitation is another property tax, payable to the local authority and collected from occupiers, whether or not they are the owners of the property. Allowances are available against both these property taxes and it is worthwhile to have the assessments checked by a professional, rather than pay them automatically by bank direct debit.

Stamp duty on purchase of a property can be substantial, although it is not charged within the five years following completion of construction when bought from the developer or on the first sale within that time limit, only a small Land Registry fee then being due.

Otherwise the rate on residential property is around 8 per cent, with small regional variations. The full rate of 17 per cent may be charged if you fail to undertake to use the land or property for this purpose within a limited time scale. Extensive grounds may be subject to a higher rate.

Value added tax (T.V.A.) is normally included in the quoted price of properties up to the age of five years. If you sell within this period you should do likewise and account for the difference in T.V.A. The rate on building land is 13 per cent and this is usually priced exclusive of T.V.A. For construction work the current rate is 18.6 per cent and again this is normally quoted *hors taxes*.

The use of offshore companies to hold property in France has diminished considerably since the introduction of stamp duty of about 20 per cent on the conveyance, plus an annual tax of 3 per cent on the capital value.

Bank accounts   Communication is all important and as many foreign banks have set up subsidiaries in France it is worthwhile investigating whether your present bank has a convenient branch. Not only can you then discuss matters more easily with the staff, but it also facilitates transfers between countries. Both current and deposit accounts are available, French withholding tax being deducted from interest on the latter as far as residents are concerned. Direct debits are known as *prélèvement* and their use in paying for utilities is recommended. The main differences which you are likely to find in French banking are that post-dated cheques are processed immediately, cheques can only be negotiated through the payee's account, bank drafts are credited only after negotiation, and the clearance procedure is slow, particularly on foreign transfers. You are only permitted to stop payment of your cheque if it has been lost or stolen. You should never attempt to withhold payment of a cheque for such reasons as failure of a tradesman to provide goods or services as agreed, because if you fail to provide funds for clearance of a cheque within fifteen days of presentation then your cheque book can be confiscated for a year and you will be debarred from opening another account.

Residence permits   Nationals of most countries can remain in France for a maximum period of three months without formalities. Obtaining a residence permit (*carte de séjour*) is not difficult. Some departments will issue the permit to EC citizens without production of a visa. Otherwise, you should visit a French consulate before leaving your home country and have a *visa de longue durée* stamped in your passport. The main requirements, apart from completing an application form, are confirmation that you have accommodation in France, that you have sufficient income on which to live and that medical cover is available, either through reciprocal arrangements for state pensioners or by means of an insurance policy. A number of passport type photographs will be required, so it is advisable to have a supply available. Fiscal stamps in payment of fees are obtainable in France from tobacconists.

Local wills The ideal arrangement for an expatriate permanently resident in France is to have a local will dealing solely with property located within France and a second will drawn in another country covering all assets situated outside of France. The main reasons for this are to reduce legal costs and to simplify the distribution of the estate on death. The charges for making wills are likely to be relatively small, whereas if there is only one will the legal costs of translation and obtaining probate in another country can be quite substantial.

It is not advisable to refrain from making any will, because if you die intestate in France then the disposal of your assets may be very different from what you may have wished. Home made wills can be very cheap, although this is often a false economy; particularly if you contravene the French laws of succession through ignorance, in which case such a will may be far worse than having none, due to the high legal costs involved in sorting out the discrepancies. French law differs from the laws of other countries and this is very noticeable in respect of the limited rights which a surviving spouse has compared with close blood relations. Protection should therefore be given by the method which you use to purchase and register your property. Even if you only have a foreign will your property in France will still be dealt with according to French law. Executors are not normally used in France, as the notary deals with the administration and distribution of the estate, as well as the arrangements for payment of inheritance tax.

ITALY

Climate Average summer temperature in the central region is 24°. The south has a mild winter and a long hot summer. Colder winters in the north, with fog. Rainfall unpredictable.

Languages Italian. Some English and French.

Travel Bureaux *Compagnia Italiana Tourismo, Piazza Repubblica 68,* Rome.

Business hours 0830-1245, 1500-1830 Monday to Friday, with regional variations. Government offices close at 1320 for the day.

Inflation 5.5 per cent.

Local banks   Banca Commerciale Italiana, Credito Italiano, Banco di Roma, Banca Nazionale del Lavoro, Banco di Napoli, Banco di Sicilia.

Precautions & problems   The interior of Sardinia and Sicily can be a little unsafe.

House purchase procedure   The procedure for buying a property in Italy is very like that in France, except that only one notary is used. Therefore, once you have found a property that appeals to you then you should immediately engage a professional adviser before you sign any document or pay over any money. The contract, called a *promessi di vendità* or a *compromesso*, is drawn up by the estate agent, frequently on the basis of only verbal information given to him by the vendor. Consequently you should insist on a full description and a plan, together with a list of fixtures and fittings being part of the contract. If you need to finance the purchase then you should ensure that a clause is inserted in the contract making it conditional upon a loan being granted, as you have this right in law. A 10 per cent deposit at this stage is general, which you should pay to the notary and not to the estate agent or vendor. Contracts are binding and the prospective purchaser forfeits the deposit if he is unable to complete, except for failure to obtain a mortgage as mentioned above. If the seller withdraws the property then he must pay twice the amount of the deposit to the prospective purchaser. Estate agents' commission rates are fixed by the *Camera di Commercio* of the locality, so it is advisable to be aware of the correct level when you check the contract, ensuring that no liability is placed upon you as a result of the vendor's failure to pay the agent. An average rate is about 5 per cent, of which the seller pays 3 per cent and the buyer 2 per cent. Your own adviser will carry out the necessary searches and advise you on progress towards completion. If you have no adviser then the notary will carry out the searches on your behalf for an extra fee, but only if you ask him to do so. Of course, you must ensure that sufficient funds are available before or on completion to pay the balance of the purchase price plus stamp duty and fees; although there is no necessity to attend in person, as you can appoint an attorney for this purpose. In any dealings regarding property, married couples should ensure that their marriage certificate is available. If you are buying a property which has an element of shared ownership you should obtain from the seller the *regolamento del condominio*, which gives the rules which you will have to observe, together with a copy of the latest account for service charges to give you a guide to expected expenses. A mortgage charge remains on the property whoever is the current owner, so you should ensure that the vendor gives an undertaking to pay it off within a limited time and you should check after a few months to confirm that this has been done. As the stamp duty alone amounts to 17 per cent you should budget for quite a large proportion of the purchase price to cover legal costs and fees.

Local mortgages First of all the warning; a foreign currency mortgage exposes you to a long term and completely open-ended currency risk and this is something which you should not undertake without proper and independent financial advice. Subsidiaries of the main banks are the usual source of property purchase loans in Italy, although the rate of interest is very likely to be excessively high. If initially the property will be used only for vacations then a maximum advance of about 60 per cent is usual, increasing to 75 per cent for one used permanently. The normal term is around fifteen years. Penalties, subject to official maxima, are likely to be imposed for early repayment and sale of the property during the term. Do not count on an inspection taking place to highlight defects, or for any insurance cover to be arranged. You are almost certainly likely to obtain better terms on a mortgage arranged in your home country.

Planning permission & building If you are purchasing land on which to build, the first point you should be aware of is that in Italy the future use of all land has already been decided and this information is contained in the records of the local *comuni*. Secondly, density zones are also fixed by the *comuni* and you will require a much larger plot in the countryside to build a big house than you would near the centre of the town. In the latter zone the proportionate size of property to land is unlikely to change, although periodic reviews may enable an extension to be built in outer zones at a later date. Finally, most building regulations are very strict and the majority of *comuni* require you to build in the local style.

The procedure is that before you purchase any land you should ensure that a new planning permission (*licenza*) is obtained, or one is already in force which preferably is not within two years of its expiry date. Although fees are likely to be about three million lire, it is advisable to have an architect or surveyor (*geometrà*) draw up plans and have them approved by the same *comuni* before committing yourself to a firm purchase of the land. This is also necessary if you are considering buying a dilapidated building for restoration. Having obtained the *licenza* and made the purchase your next step is to conclude a contract with a builder to carry out the necessary work, ensuring that substantial penalties for late completion are provided for. Supervision of the contract will be undertaken by your architect or suveyor, for which the normal fee is about 5 to 10 per cent of the building cost. Their certificates should be obtained before making periodical stage payments. Generally they can be left to oversee matters, although you should make a personal check that the thickness of the insulation is likely to meet your needs. The rate of value added tax (I.V.A.) in Italy on new building work is 19 per cent and you should ensure that the bill for construction work itemises this separately.

On completion of the construction it is examined by an official of the *comune* and if the property meets the requirements regarding strength, allowed dimensions and other matters, then a document called a *collaudo* will be issued at a cost of up to 300,000 lire. This enables you to obtain a habitation certificate from the town hall. Connection of electricity, water and possibly gas in town can then be arranged.

Utilities, costs and maintenance   Mains water is invariably drinkable. If you have your own supply it will be tested occasionally at your expense. During the summer months curtailment of supply should be expected in all areas south of the valley of the River Po at times. In view of this, installation of a tank for domestic supply should be considered, with possibly another for garden use, both being subject to official permission. The problem is more severe in country areas and here you are likely to require a pump to provide sufficient pressure to operate a water heater. You should establish at the earliest opportunity your entitlement to local water sources including wells, besides discovering who else has the right to use your source. Swimming pools invariably require planning permission. If you do not have mains drainage be certain that you know the location of the septic tank and the procedure for arranging its emptying. A separate septic tank will be needed for a swimming pool. Water costs in Italy are around 1,230 lire per cubic metre, probably the third highest in the world.

E.N.E.L. is the monopoly supplier of electricity in Italy at 230 volts AC. Normal supply is only three kilowatts and higher can only be obtained with a special contract and an increased standing charge. Electricity costs per kWh are a fair amount higher than in France and Britain. Installation in a very remote area may well cost about 4 million lire, although if there is already a supply to nearby properties then 400,000 lire is a more likely figure in the countryside. Consumption is charged bi-monthly, estimates being used except in June and December. Payment can be made by cheque or at the post office. However, if you are likely to be absent, direct debit arrangements are advisable, as reconnection is very slow. Even if you do pay your bills promptly continuity of supply is often suspect.

Mains gas may well be advisable in urban locations. If not and elsewhere, bottled gas is widely used for cooking and possibly for water heating, although a gas tank is often fitted for the latter purpose.

Central heating is cheapest when it is run on mains gas, the best alternatives being oil, electricity and gas tanks in that order of priority.

Società Italiana per l'Esercizio delle Telecomunicazioni (S.I.P.) has almost a monopoly of domestic telephone business. Except in some large cities installation of a telephone is not generally subject to a long delay. A doctor's support will give you priority for medical reasons. Connection charges in towns are low, although they can be as high as 200,000 lire in a remote area for a new installation. Ordinary tariff applies from 0800-0830 and 1330-1830 on weekdays, 0800-1300 on Saturdays and costs about 30 per cent more than in Britain. There is a surcharge of 40 per cent on all calls made between 0830 and 1330 on weekdays. The evening rate is effective from 1830 to 2200 and the lowest rate applies from then until 0800. Bills are rendered bi-monthly, which you can pay in cash at a post office or S.I.P. office, by cheque to your area office, or by bank direct debit. The latter is recommended. It is extremely expensive to obtain equipment on hire purchase from S.I.P. Purchases from other sources require the approval of S.I.P.

Rubbish collection and the water rates are covered by a local tax which is mentioned later. There will be community or service charges if you own common property. Insurance is available underwritten by Lloyds of London for a premium of £2 per £1000 on buildings and £6 per £1000 on contents, the policy covering earthquakes, which Italian companies exclude. There are many other exclusions on Italian policies which you would normally expect to be included, such as damage caused by burst water pipes for instance. In wooded areas the fire risk is very serious and you should keep your grounds clear of dry material on pain of a heavy fine for neglect. Maintenance costs for external decoration will rise from south to north due to very different weather conditions. There will also be variations in charges approximately in line with property values.

Common property If there is an element of shared ownership which goes with the property, such as common staircases, roof space, swimming pool, etc., and there are at least five co-owners of a block of flats or other property, then it is necessary under Italian law to form an *ente condominiale*. The law specifies that rules must be drawn up in a *Regolamento del condominio*, which covers the appointment of an *amministratore*, holding of meetings of owners, management of the block, calculation of the share of service charges, what is permitted and what is prohibited, as well as other relevant matters. The rules have the force of law and they must be within a specified framework.

An Annual General Meeting is obligatory every year to appoint an *amministratore*, possibly assisted by a committee, to approve the budget and to deal with any other business of the *condominio*. The proceedings take place in Italian. You are entitled to appoint a proxy to attend meetings (even if you are in residence) and it may be advisable to do so in order to protect your interests. Service charges are normally collected in two instalments. A prospective buyer is entitled to ask for a copy of the last account, as well as the rules.

Taxes   Every individual's tax situation is different with various income levels and allowances available, so it is not possible to tell you exactly how much income tax you will pay if you go to live in Italy. However, the fiscal year commences on 1 January and you will be liable for income tax (*Imposte sui Redditi delle Pensone Fisiche* or I.R.P.E.F.) if you are resident in Italy for more than 183 days in total in a calendar year. You are exempted from filing an income tax return if you have no income, or it consists only of state pensions, voluntary payments, capital transfers, capital gains (other than on property sales), or gambling proceeds. Not later than the end of May others must file their return and pay any tax due. Subsequent to the first return it is necessary to pay 95 per cent of the tax previously paid by the end of November. Due to the enormous fines for incorrect declarations you are advised to engage a *commercialistà* to file your return for a small fee. Those with a particularly high income may like to know that the top rate of income tax is 53 per cent, which is much higher than in most European countries. Italy has double taxation treaties with many other states and if you have paid income tax in your country of origin then it is very likely that you will able to deduct this sum from Italian tax due.

On every sale of real property without exception *Imposta Comunale sull' Incremento del Valore degli Immobili* (I.N.V.I.M.), a capital gains tax, is levied and is payable to the local *comune*. The minimum rate is 3 per cent and the maximum 30 per cent, the latter applying on a profit on sale exceeding 200 per cent. The tax is not levied on other types of capital gains at present.

Imposte di successione (inheritance tax) is payable at death by the beneficiaries, including the surviving spouse, on a scale and at a rate according to the closeness of the relationship. Estates valued at less than 30 million lire are exempted. The maximum rate between parents and children is 31 per cent on a bequest of 1,000 million lire. For unrelated persons the rate is 60 per cent at that amount.

Imposte Locale sui Reditti (I.L.O.R.) is a local tax to cover garbage collection and water rates. Depending upon your level of income and the size of your house it varies between a minimum of 40,000 lire and a maximum of 400,000 lire. Non-residents are also due to pay this tax. Residents can deduct the amount paid against their income tax liability.

Stamp duty is charged on the purchase of houses and apartments at 10 per cent. On land it is assessed at 17 per cent. Local density zoning regulations will decide the amount of surplus to be charged at the higher rate for houses and some apartments having their own grounds. It is important not to accept an understated value for this purpose on buying property, because by so doing you leave yourself open to a much higher capital gains tax assessment at 30 per cent in the apparent profit on sale.

Imposta sul Valore Aggiunto (I.V.A.) is a value added tax which Italy as an EC country is obliged to charge. At present it is levied at 9 per cent on food, 19 per cent on building work and at higher levels for luxuries. When you receive an estimate to build or reconstruct your property check whether it includes I.V.A., as it is more usual to quote an exclusive price.

Bank accounts   Exchange control is being dismantled in Italy and most if not all of the regulations should disappear in the near future, although the process is subject to almost daily changes. It is advisable to enquire from friends and neighbours which banks speak languages which you understand and are not excessively inefficient. Expect transfers from other countries to take about three weeks in transit and for cheques which you draw to be delayed in presentation. Interest on deposit accounts is subject to withholding tax in the case of residents. It is advisable to use the direct debit system for paying bills of utilities, as immediate disconnection swiftly follows the expiry of the final date for payment. Post-dated cheques are cleared when they are presented. It is not advisable to have your cheque unpaid for more than fifteen days, as legal proceedings follow and you may well be prohibited from holding a bank account in the future. Certified cheques (*assegno circolare*) can be obtained from banks at low cost, although you should ensure their security and treat them as cash.

Residence permits   Most foreigners are allowed to stay in Italy for at least three months and however long you intend to remain your first step should be to complete a *Dichiarazione di Soggiorno per Stranieri* at the local *comune* offices. Before this expires you should renew it with the local *carabinieri* if you reside in the countryside, or alternatively with the *Polizia di Stato*. Various questions will be asked of you, including your income level, depending upon the area; although little documentation is likely to be required apart from confirmation that you are covered by reciprocal health agreements, or that you have private medical insurance. Besides your passport you will need to supply three photographs and probably a *carta bollata* costing 5,000 lire from tobacconists. The *soggiorno* normally lasts for five years before requiring renewal. When driving a vehicle it is obligatory to carry identification.

Local wills   There are a lot of variables regarding what will happen to your estate at your death depending upon whether you die intestate, have only an Italian will, only a will made in your country of origin, or wills made in both countries. Also the position is complicated by whether your assets are all situated in Italy, some in your home country, or possibly some in a third country. Two things are certain: do not write a home made will in Italy and do not leave your will in an Italian bank safety deposit box, as access is impossible at death until the estate is settled and proved. In complicated circumstances you are advised to engage an *avvocato*, although you can go directly to a notary to make an Italian will. A foreign will is acted upon in Italy, although you should be aware that translation and legalization costs are likely to be fairly high. For this reason it is usually advisable to have an Italian will covering your property and assets situated in Italy. Whether you also make a will in your home country covering the remainder of the estate will probably depend upon whether that country has higher or lower inheritance taxes than Italy. For instance, surviving spouses are exempted from this tax in the UK and there is exemption up to a fairly high threshold. Conversely, the highest rate can be 40 per cent in Britain, although the maximum is 31 per cent for close relations in Italy on estates valued over 1,000 million lire. Remember that Italian law protects the inheritance of children and they cannot be excluded from benefit under an Italian will.

MALTA

Climate   Most rain is confined to the winter and spring. Temperature rises gradually from 10°C to 21°C in January and February to 25°C to 31°C in July to September, occasionally 38°C. Humid in summer.

Languages   Maltese and English. Italian often understood.

Social customs   Dress is generally rather formal.

Travel Bureaux   National Tourist Organisation, The Palace, Valletta.

Local maps   Obtain from foreign suppliers.

Business hours   0830-1245, 1430-1730 Monday to Friday. 0830-1300 Saturday.

Inflation   1.3 per cent.

Local banks   Bank of Valletta Ltd, Mid-Med Bank Ltd, Lombard Bank (Malta) Ltd.

Precautions & problems   When living in Malta for a number of years I found the main difficulty was the rather claustrophobic feeling of being on fairly small islands which you could only leave by air or sea. The attraction for expatriates is likely to vary according to which political party is in power. Driving standards are abysmal in high density traffic. During and after rain treat the slippery roads as if they were covered in ice.

House purchase procedure Advertisements appear in the daily newspaper *Malta Times*, which is published in English. There are a number of estate agents in Malta and local property is also handled by agents in other countries, such as Malta Property Consultants Ltd, 22 Vicarage Hill, Farnham, Surrey GU9 8HJ, England. A preliminary agreement is signed which is binding on both parties and a 10 per cent deposit is paid; withdrawal being possible in the case of a faulty title or non-issue of government permits. The property must be valued at a minimum of 15,000 Maltese lira (about £26,000 sterling), although the renovation costs of a dilapidated property can be included. Most sales are on a perpetual leasehold basis, but the freehold can often be purchased for twenty times the annual ground rent. A Maltese notary handles the applications for government permits, as well as conducting the searches, for a fee of 1 per cent of contract value. The Ministry of Finance fee is about £175 sterling and stamp duty is 13.55 per cent. Leasehold properties attract a fee equivalent to one year's ground rent.

Local mortgages The usual warning must be given that this involves an open-ended currency risk as described in Chapter 6. In such a small and undiversified economy as Malta the currency must be expected to have wide fluctuations. Maltese banks offer loans for a period of three to five years, the interest only being paid during the term of the loan. A guarantee from a foreign bank secured on an overseas property is required as collateral for the loan. The present interest rate is 8 per cent. Only on Gozo (the second largest island) Malta Property Consultants offer 50 per cent mortgages for five years secured upon a Gozo property at about the same rate of interest.

Planning permission & building A permit to construct a new building is almost impossible to obtain, as the Maltese authorities do not wish to spoil the appearance of the islands with ugly modern architecture. However, there should be no problem in obtaining permission for renovation work providing that it blends in with the local style. Maltese builders and carpenters are expert craftsmen.

Utilities, costs & maintenance Malta has a low cost of living index assessed at 86.6, compared with 100 for London, 93.4 for Berlin, 101.7 for Paris, 110.0 for Geneva, 124.2 for Stockholm and 129 for Oslo.

Taxes   The taxation of expatriates depends upon their residence status (see also as follows under *'Residence permits'*). Non-residents are not taxed providing that their stay in Malta does not exceed three months in a continuous period, or six months in total during a fiscal year.

'Temporary residents' (so called, although their stay may in fact be permanent) are taxed if they remain in Malta for a continuous period of at least six months, but only on their remittances to the Maltese Islands. The rate of tax is calculated on a sliding scale between a minimum of 10 per cent and a maximum of 35 per cent.

Permanent residents, who must have a global income of at least the equivalent of LM 10,000 (about £17,500) per annum, or global capital to a minimum value of LM 150,000 (around £262,000), are required to remit to Malta not less than LM 6,000 for a single person plus LM 1,000 for each dependant. Tax is assessed only on such remittances (less personal allowances) at a rate of 15 per cent, subject to a minimum tax of LM 1,000.

Bank accounts   These present no problems for most of the local expatriates because all of the staff of banks speak English and documentation is in that language. Banks are closed on quite a few days during a year, as there are many fiestas.

Residence permits   Most nationals arriving on the islands require no further documentation for a stay of up to three months other than the entry visa, which is granted automatically to most visitors on arrival.

The vast majority who wish to remain for a longer period opt for 'temporary resident' status, mainly because they are unable to meet the requirements of a high income or substantial capital needed for 'permanent resident' status. However, the former presents no obstacle to permanent residence in fact. To obtain temporary residence it is only necessary to produce proof of an adequate income to the immigration authorities and the entry visa can be renewed each year.

'Permanent resident' status includes entitlement to free treatment in Maltese hospitals. To achieve it you only need to demonstrate to the immigration authorities documentary evidence of global income of at least the equivalent of LM 10,000 per annum, or global capital to a minimum value of LM 150,000. Remittances to Malta must be not less than the equivalent of LM 6,000 for a single person plus LM 1,000 for each dependant. Consequently, a married couple with no resident children would need to transfer just over £12,000 sterling each year at present.

Local wills   It is advisable to have local wills covering assets situated in Malta and this is easily arranged through a local lawyer. A 'quick succession' clause, as mentioned in Chapter 24, is advisable in view of local traffic conditions in case husband and wife both die shortly after an accident.

PORTUGAL

Climate Peninsula: Most rain falls in winter, heaviest in the north-west. The south has moderate winters and long hot summers. The north-west has moderate winters and short summers. The north-east has long, cold winters and hot summers.

Madeira: Sub-tropical. July and August are the hottest and most humid months; November to March the wettest.

Azores: Wet winters, with violent gales. Hot and humid in July and August.

Languages Portuguese. Some Spanish, English and French.

Social customs Much formality and courtesy.

Travel bureaux National Tourist Office, *S.E.I.T., Palacio Faz, Praça dos Restauradores,* Lisbon.

Local maps Generally available.

Business hours 0900-1300, 1500-1900 (1730 in Madeira) Monday to Friday. 0900-1300 Saturday.

Inflation 10.2 per cent.

Local banks *Banco Espirito Santo e Comercial de Lisboa, Banco Totta & Açores, Banco Portugues de Atlantico,* Bank of London and South America.

Precautions & problems Although the cost of living is relatively low, inflation is quite high and likely to remain in double figures in the near future. Exchange control should be expected to remain in force until 1995.

House purchase procedure You have a number of methods open to you when you decide to seek a property in Portugal. You can visit a local estate agent, although they do not exist in all areas. Remember that they may be attempting to force the price up to the highest level as the excess is their commission, or they may be selling some properties which they own. You could contact a property developer either in Portugal or perhaps in your home country, where exhibitions may well be held. Finally, there are various expatriate newspapers printed in Portugal with a wide range of resale properties available. Having discovered one which appeals to you the first sensible step which you should take, before you sign anything or pay any money, is to engage a local professional adviser, or you may lose a large sum and end up with nothing. Although in theory you could do much of the necessary checking yourself, if you are not fluent in Portuguese or do not understand the legal significance of certain facts then you are well advised to find an *advogado* who speaks your language or has a multilingual staff. Then it is usual to commence by signing a reservation, accompanied by a small returnable deposit. The land registry is next searched to check that there is a good title, as well as no mortgages, charges or restrictive covenants. The local tax office register also needs to be checked to confirm that property taxes have been paid and that the details are identical to the land registry. In the case of a new building you should confirm that the necessary permits and licences are in order and that the builder has complied with planning rules. Your lawyer will then agree that you may sign the *contrato de promessa de compra e venda* if the above matters are in order. Strictly speaking you could be sued to complete if you attempted to withdraw after signing the binding contract, although there would be little chance of enforcement if your assets were abroad. Naturally, you would lose your deposit. Similarly, if the vendor withdrew the property subsequently you could sue for completion. However, in view of the very slow process of actions through the courts you would probably be well advised to accept the usual penalty of double the amount of your deposit. As long as exchange control regulations are in force (probably until 1995) the next step is to submit the appropriate form to the Bank of Portugal applying for an import licence for foreign currency. Then go to the local tax office to apply for your tax card with a fiscal number and pay the conveyancing tax called S.I.S.A. (see details under 'taxes' following) or make a claim for exemption. When the import licence is received vendor and purchaser (in person, or power of attorney can be given to another) go to the notary and the *escritura* (deed) is written and signed. It is then essential for the *escritura* to be taken to the local land registry with the absolute minimum of delay, or someone else may be registered as owner of the property in priority to you. The last step is to register with the local tax office for payment of local rates. It is advisable to allow up to 20 per cent of the purchase price for legal costs, taxes, registration fees and other costs.

Local mortgages   Two warnings on this subject. Firstly, consider with extreme care the completely open-ended currency risk which this involves, explained in Chapter 6. The escudo has just entered the European Monetary System, so there is a limit to possible fluctuations.

Secondly, Portugal has inflation in double figures and high interest rates go hand in hand with high inflation, consequently the interest on a mortgage expressed in escudos is likely to cost you more than obtaining one in your own country. There are also advantages of simplification in selling if your mortgage has not been granted in Portugal. That said, if you still wish to obtain a mortgage in Portugal then your first step should be to contact your Portuguese bank, as they all have their own rules. Alternatively, if you own properties in two countries, you may find it relatively simple to obtain a second mortgage secured on the one you own in your home country to enable you to purchase a Portuguese property. UK tax residents should obtain competent professional advice and be careful that they do not disturb their present mortgage relief arrangements on income tax. Also that they protect themselves by ensuring the loan agreement confirms that the interest rate payable is after deduction of UK withholding tax if a foreign bank is involved, other than one resident in the UK. British residents may like to know that a mortgage secured on a Portuguese property can be obtained in the UK from the following banks:

> *Banco Espirito Santo e Comercial de Lisboa,*
> 4, Fenchurch Street, London EC3
> *Banco Portugues do Atlantico,*
> 77 Gracechurch Street, London EC3
> *Banco Totta & Açores,*
> 68 Cannon Street, London EC4

Other nationals may well find that similar arrangements are available in their own country.

Planning permission & building You would be extremely unwise in Portugal to obtain planning permission and negotiate a building contract yourself without competent professional legal advice. However, an outline of the necessary steps are as follows. In this connection land is divided into one of three groups: agricultural, rustic or a *loteamento* (building plot). In the case of the first two it is necessary to obtain the permission of the Ministry of Agriculture and additionally in the case of agricultural land you will need to confirm that you intend to farm it and produce evidence of the necessary experience. It is then advisable to apply to the *Camara* (town hall) for outline planning permission before you purchase the land. If you are dealing with a developer and building has not yet commenced on the plot, then you should insist on buying the plot before construction commences as a separate operation in order to protect your interests. Obtain legal advice before signing any document purported to be merely a reservation of a plot and ensure that any deposit is returnable. Similarly, your solicitor should approve the terms of the contract and ensure that you are fully protected in such matters as supply of utilities etc. It is also necessary to check that the developer actually has detailed planning permission.

If no developer is involved you will need to find a reliable and competent architect to prepare plans to your liking, draw up the bill of quantities, deal with infrastructure requirements and make the application for detailed planning permission. When the building permit is received the next step is to select someone to do the construction work and to agree on a building contract. Do not accept a 'take it or leave it' attitude from the first builder you contact, as this may well be an indication of his unreliability. Certainly you should insist on a penalty clause for late completion assessed on an ongoing basis. Stage payments should be due as phases are completed on your architect's certificates. A good solicitor will give you sound advice on the various matters on which you should protect yourself, as much can go wrong. The absolute minimum is that the contract should contain a clause to the effect that all matters not specifically covered are subject to the provisions of the Portuguese Civil Code, as the absence of this proviso may well mean that you are signing away your legal rights in the event of a dispute. On completion it is essential to exercise your right to an inspection, either in person or better still by a professional, otherwise your entitlement to rectification of defects could well be lost. On acceptance the property is inspected by an official from the town hall, who completes a certificate of habitation if he is satisfied. This document is used to arrange connection to the electricity supply. It is also taken to the Land Registry to obtain the land registration certificate and to the local tax office for the fiscal document called the *caderneta predial*.

Utilities, costs and maintenance   Hard water is the norm in most of Portugal and you should be prepared to deal with problems in the system caused by scale. In a number of coastal locations in the southern half of the country the water often becomes rather brackish as the dry summer progresses. Continuity of supply in this area is uncertain, leading to the expense of buying bottled water. On urbanizations mains supply is normal, but in the countryside you may depend upon a well, so it is important to establish who owns it and who has access. Local authority permission is required for a large cistern. Besides a standing charge, water is metered and consumption is invoiced. There is no monopoly supplier of water throughout the country, so costs do vary and can be high for connection from a private company.

On an urbanization it is usual to pay only for an electricity contract and the meter. Elsewhere the charge for connection to the supply could be very substantial indeed, particularly if your property is in an isolated location. Direct debit is the best method of payment to ensure that you do not have the expense of a reconnection charge following discontinuance due to an unpaid bill.

Bottled gas is a very useful alternative to using electricity for water heating, cooking and space heating. Ensure adequate ventilation.

Mains drainage is common in coastal urbanizations built in recent years. In the countryside it is much more normal to find that you have a septic tank. Make certain that you know where the covers are situated and enquire about the arrangements for emptying it. In some cases this is the responsibility of the local authority, for which a tax is levied.

If you wish to have a telephone installed it is a simple matter to contact the company for a quotation. On acceptance delay in installation may not be excessive if lines are available. If not, you may well have to wait for years. Should the telephone be required for business or medical reasons then priority can often be obtained with the necessary documentary confirmation.

For those who live in an apartment or on an urbanization where there are shared facilities there will be a community charge to pay, which you can discover before deciding to purchase. Rates will also be payable, the amount being known to the previous owner in the case of a resale, or otherwise the local authorities will advise you. Building and contents insurance is essential. You may well find that Portuguese policies exclude claims for important matters such as theft and burst water pipes. Good cover is available underwritten by Lloyds of London for a premium of £2 per £1000 for buildings and £6 per £1000 for contents, the policy being in English. Finally, remember that there will be maintenance costs because, although you do not have the level of urban pollution found in northern Europe, the fact that buildings are painted a light colour entails repainting at intervals. The salt in sea breezes will have an effect upon metalwork in coastal areas.

Common property   In Portugal when you buy an apartment with its own entrance you do so freehold. A deed of horizontal property is constituted to regulate the maintenance of common areas such as staircases, roof, swimming pools, green areas, patios, garages and parking spaces. An annual general meeting is called in the first month of every year to approve past expenditure, agree a budget and appoint an administrator for two years, possibly assisted by a committee. Owners are charged a proportion of the expenses in an agreed formula. Purchasers are entitled to see the deed so that they can understand their rights and liabilities, as well as have a copy of the last community charge account. Buyers of such property are advised for their own protection to check whether the developer has obtained a mortgage upon the whole building and, if so, to insist upon bank confirmation that such mortgage will be released on the date you complete your purchase.

Taxes Taking firstly Portuguese income tax (*Imposto Sobre o Rendimento das Pessoas Singulares*), you are liable for this as a resident if either (a) you own a property in Portugal on the last day of the calendar year with the intention of making it your home, however many days you spend in it; or (b) you are present in Portugal for at least a total of 183 days (not necessarily consecutive) in a calendar year. As a resident your global income will be assessed and charged on the following basis:

CHARGEABLE INCOME   PERCENTAGE

Escudos	Excess	Rate
Up to 450,000	16	16
450,000-850,000	20	17.882
850,000-1,250,000	27.5	20.96
1,250,000-3,000,000	35	29.15
Above 3,000,000	40	

The calculations are done by taking the rate percentage for the next lower income band than your own on the maximum figure of that band and adding any additional amount at the excess percentage shown for your band. Example: On a chargeable income of 1,000,000 escudos tax is:

850,000 @ 17.882%	=	151,997 escudos
150,000 @ 27.5%	=	41,250 escudos
Total income tax due	=	193,247 escudos

Special arrangements apply to pensioners, as no tax is charged on pensions not exceeding 400,000 escudos per annum. For pensions between 400,000 and 1,000,000 escudos a deduction of 400,000 escudos is allowed and only 50 per cent of the excess is charged.

Interest on investments and desposits is charged at 20 per cent. This book is mainly concerned with retirement abroad, although income of non-residents is generally assessed at a flat rate of 25 per cent.

Capital gains tax is payable by both residents and non-residents on gains arising from (a) share transfers or sales of personal property (b) sales of real property and (c) premiums received on assigning leases or rental agreements. Property (but not building land) acquired in 1988 or earlier is exempted. The gain is indexed for inflation over periods exceeding two years and only the excess is charged. This latter figure is regarded as additional income in the year of assessment and it is charged at 50 per cent of the normal income tax rate.

Portuguese inheritance tax is levied on both resident and non-resident beneficiaries, including the surviving spouse in both categories. Non-residents are charged only on assets situated in Portugal; but in the case of residents it is assessed on global property. Calculation is a little complicated because relationships to the deceased are firstly split into four groups:

Class I	–	spouse and children (including adopted) under 21 years.
Class II	–	other children and grandchildren.
Class III	–	brothers, sisters, parents and grandparents.
Class IV	–	other relatives and unrelated.

The taxable value (not the market value) is then charged according to the following table:

Escudos		*Class*		
	I	II	III	IV
	%	%	%	%
100,000-250,000	–	4	10	30
250,000-500,000	8	10	16	38
500,000-1,000,000	13	16	23	46
1,000,000-5,000,000	18	21	29	53
5,000,000-10,000,000	23	26	36	60
10,000,000-50,000,000	33	36	49	76

After deciding upon the class of relationship take the percentage on the maximum limit for the band below the bequest and add the percentage on the excess at the rate for the total bequest band.
Example: Property left to a surviving spouse is valued at 15 times fiscal letting value = 50,000 escudos × 15 = 750,000 escudos. Relationship is Class I.

500,000 escudos @ 8%	=	40,000 escudos
250,000 escudos @ 13%	=	32,500 escudos
Inheritance tax due	=	72,500 escudos

This is collected by half yearly instalments over a period of thirty-six months. There is a discount for early payment on a sliding scale of up to 30 per cent.

S.I.S.A. is a tax on the conveyance of real estate from one owner to another. On residential property it is levied at 5 per cent of the official value when the latter exceeds 7.6 million escudos and at 10 per cent above 22.8 million escudos. A sliding scale operates between these two figures. Rustic land being sold attracts an 8 per cent rate. For buildings and building land the charge is assessed at 10 per cent. There are likely to be very serious financial consequences if you understate values for S.I.S.A. purposes, so do not agree to such a suggestion by the vendor.

There is now a municipal tax (*contribuição autarquica*) of about 1.2 per cent of fiscal value on urban properties. The component parts of mixed properties are valued separately and taxed at the appropriate rates. Permanent residents are exempted from this tax provided (a) they occupy the property for at least ten years (b) the fiscal value is less than 10 million escudos and (c) they move in within six months of purchase unless circumstances prevent them from doing so.

Finally, as with any EC country, there is a value added tax (I.V.A.). It is levied at various rates depending upon the class of goods or services. For building contracts it is assessed at 17 per cent and you should check whether you are being quoted an I.V.A. inclusive price, as payment is your responsibility.

Bank accounts　　The first point to remember is that there is exchange control in Portugal and the EC has agreed that it may continue to restrict transactions until 1995. When bringing money into Portugal to buy a property you should invariably obtain an import licence. Similarly on a sale, an export licence is required to repatriate the proceeds. When you first move to Portugal you are allowed to have both non-resident escudo and foreign currency accounts. One year after the date on which your residence permit is issued you are no longer permitted to operate the above accounts and the only type of account you may hold is a resident escudo account. Current and deposit accounts are available, withholding tax being deducted from interest on the latter at 20 per cent. A non-resident can bring into Portugal unlimited amounts of foreign currency plus a maximum of 50,000 escudos. Residents are limited to the same amount of escudos plus the equivalent of 150,000 escudos in foreign currency. On leaving the country you can carry 50,000 escudos, but proof of importation will be needed if a larger sum is involved.

Residence permits　　Most of the preparatory authorization is done in your home country and as it takes a considerable amount of time it is advisable to make the application for a visa at the very earliest opportunity. This is done by submitting form V-2 to your Portuguese consulate together with certain information and quite a number of documents, the regulations being subject to variation, particularly with the advent of full membership of the EC.

Pensioners should have no difficulties, although others will have to produce evidence of sufficient means. This visa is valid for a maximum period of 120 days. You still have to apply for a residence permit within 90 days after your arrival in Portugal at a foreigners' department

(*Servicos de Estrangeiros*) of the local office of the Ministry of Internal Affairs to be found in most larger towns. Apart from having a visa, retired people will only need to complete a questionnaire and supply a certificate of registration with their consulate together with their latest bank statement. During your first five years in Portugal a renewable permit is normally applied for annually.

Local wills   You can prepare a will in your handwriting and in your own language to pass it to a Portuguese notary for authentication but not notation, although it is advisable to have legal assistance in its drafting. The alternative is to have a will prepared written in Portuguese, possibly by your local lawyer, to have notarised and entered in the official records. In any case it is advisable to have some kind of local will, probably covering assets situated in Portugal, as proving foreign wills is lengthy and expensive. To reduce costs it is probably advisable to appoint a Portuguese lawyer as executor and to agree to professional charges.

SPAIN

Climate   Peninsula: Temperate in the north. Dry, hot summers in other regions. Central area is very cold from December to March with night minimum often not far above freezing. The south and east have very mild winters, with a high proportion of sunny days.

Canaries: Warm and dry for most of the year. Average temperatures are 17°C in winter, 22°C in summer.
Balearics: Very similar to the eastern coastal region of the peninsula.

Languages   Spanish; Catalan in the east and Balearics; Basque in the Pyrenees. Some English and French is understood.

Social customs   Late lunch and evening meal. Time has little meaning to Spaniards and it is unwise to rely upon firm appointments.

Travel bureaux   There are national and provincial tourist offices in most large towns, the standard of service being very variable.

Local maps   *Instituto Geografico Nacional, General Ibáñez de Ibero, 3, 28003 Madrid.* Telephone 233 3800.

Business hours   Mostly commence at 0900, but vary considerably according to locality and season. Afternoon siesta is widespread, with evening opening.

Inflation   Officially 6.5 per cent, although expatriates should treat this figure with caution.

Local banks   A great many foreign banks, besides national banks, regional banks and savings banks. Recommendations therefore depend upon area and local expatriate advice should be sought.

Precautions & problems   Spain can be (and often is) a very noisy place, both by day and by night, so if this bothers you then you should select your retirement location with great care. There is a widespread security problem and adequate protection should be fitted to your property.

House purchase procedure   It is not difficult to find suitable accommodation at a reasonable price, whether it is new or resale. In Spain there are many estate agencies, as well as expatriate newspapers such as *The Entertainer* covering most regions of the costas, and others like the *Costa Blanca News* or the *Weekly Post* specific to a certain area all carrying many property advertisements. Property developers have local offices, besides organizing exhibitions in and arranging inspection flights from a number of European countries. When you have discovered a property which suits you it is advisable to conclude a preliminary agreement stating that the deposit is returnable if the title is defective or if the vendor does not proceed to completion. Purchasers should always engage a lawyer (*abogado*), who is not also acting for the seller, to look after their interests in such ways as ensuring that the contract is fair to them, that the property has a clear title, there are no charges or arrears of mortgage payments and that public works are not planned through or near the property, besides private building in the vicinity which could detract from the enjoyment. When these formalities have been completed the final step evidencing ownership is for the vendor and purchaser (in person, or by power of attorney) to appear before a *notario* to sign an *escritura de compraventa* (the deeds). Details of the latter should be entered in the property register without delay, as only then is your title to the property complete and protected against creditors' liens against the vendor. All money imported into the country by non-residents for the purpose of property purchase should be paid into a non-resident account with a Spanish bank, a certificate to this effect being obtained and incorporated into your *escritura*. Strictly speaking the legal position in Spain is that the vendor is responsible for the *plus valía* tax and the *notario's* fees, whereas the buyer is liable for the transfer tax and the registration fees besides, of course, the charges of his own lawyer. Often if the contract is drawn up by the seller's lawyer then the purchaser is made responsible for all charges (*todos gastos*). It is a matter of negotiation whether the latter agrees to this arrangement. As a result of the above you should budget for between a minimum of 8 per cent and a maximum of 12 per cent of the purchase price for your costs depending upon which charges you accept, *plus valía* tax being rather variable in amount as detailed below.

Local mortgages Mortgages expressed in pesetas are not recommended at present. Not only are local interest rates extremely high, but this currency must be expected to fluctuate within wide limits for which you are responsible. For instance, the peseta recently appreciated against sterling by 16 per cent in one year and although both currencies are now in the European Monetary System they can still diverge by 12 per cent, apart from any devaluation. Consequently a second mortgage raised on a foreign property expressed in the currency in which your income arises is a better alternative. However, if you must have a local mortgage a number of options are open to a Spanish resident and rather fewer to non-residents. For example, a UK resident can only obtain a loan from a Spanish bank if certain conditions are met, such as it being for the purchase of a new property from a Spanish national. Generally it is restricted to 50 per cent of value and repayable between three and ten years. For those resident in Spain the limit may be 70 or 80 per cent and the term extended up to twenty years. Loans may be obtained from branches of Spanish banks established abroad. They can also be raised on the security of Spanish property from foreign banks and financial institutions, such as certain building societies.

Planning permission & building Although there is no reason why you should not engage your own architect or builder to construct a property on building land which you have purchased, the vast majority of expatriates buying new property in Spain obtain it from a promoter, as most construction proceeds through this means. If you take the former course legal advice is necessary right from the initial point of acquiring the land. You will need professional assistance to obtain all the necessary permits and permissions, as Spanish bureaucracy is extremely lengthy and involved. When construction is complete a Habitation Certificate (*Cedula de Habitabilidad*) must be sought. This in turn enables you to obtain a Certificate of Electrical Installation (*Bolétin de Instalaciones Eléctricas*) and a Certificate of Completion of Work (*Certificado de Fin de Obra*). If you buy through a developer then the company will obtain all these documents, which are essential to obtain a supply of electricity, water and gas. Whichever your method of acquiring a new property, stage payments are normal and you should bear in mind the implicit currency risk if you are buying in pesetas over an extended period. Wherever possible attempt to link stage payments to building progress rather than time scales and try to negotiate an ongoing penalty clause for late completion.

Utilities, costs and maintenance   The documents necessary to obtain connection to services in the first instance are mentioned above. In the case of resales it is essential to obtain the previous electricity, water and gas contracts so that the new owners can be registered.

Water in some areas may have antibodies which take a little time to get used to at first, although invariably it is drinkable. Much water is pumped from underground supplies without any trace of salinity and rivers are dammed throughout Spain to provide surface supplies. Generally continuity of supply is good in most areas, even through the normal summer drought. Scale can often impair the efficiency of electric kettles and gas water heaters, so you should be prepared to deal with this problem at intervals. Water is metered and charged every two months. Costs vary according to suppliers in various locations and a differential rate is often charged for consumption above a minimum level. However, typical costs are 40 to 52 pesetas per cubic litre, so you should budget for at least 4,500 pesetas per year including standing charges and value added tax when one person occupies a property alone and around 6,000 pesetas per annum per person for larger households. Naturally, a swimming pool will add to your costs.

Iberdrola, although not a monopoly, is the main supplier of electricity at 220 or 225 volts AC, although it may be 110 volts in parts of the Balearic Islands. Usually there is no difficulty in obtaining a supply fairly promptly, even in most country areas. Normal demand is only 3 kilowatts (which is equivalent to three bars on an electric fire), which can cause continuous problems if you cook by electricity. Supply can be increased, although this involves a higher standing charge. A typical budget cannot be suggested as this will depend upon whether you use electricity for water heating, cooking or space heating. However, in addition to a standing charge of about 1,500 pesetas every two months for normal supply, the cost is around 13 pesetas per kWh plus 12 per cent value added tax on both. Payment by bank debit is advised to avoid a reconnection charge. It is usual for alternate bills to be based upon an estimated consumption.

Bottled gas is widely used throughout the country because the cost is so cheap at around 800 pesetas per cylinder. It is also much more economical to use than electricity for heating purposes in a gas fire. Opinions vary regarding its use for water heating and perhaps the decision depends upon the quantity of hot water you use and whether a fairly continuous supply is necessary. Local experts say that you should expect problems with scale in gas water heaters. Cooking with gas obviates the maximum demand problems of electricity, besides being considerably cheaper.

Mains drainage is generally part of the infrastructure of urbanizations built in recent years. This may well not be the case in the countryside, where septic tanks are widely used.

Delays in waiting for the installation of a telephone in Spain from the monopoly supplier *Telefonica* are some of the longest of any country in Europe, frequently being measured in years rather than months. Consequently, you should make a written application at the earliest opportunity. This does not commit you to accept the quotation eventually received. No estimate of installation costs can be given here as it depends upon numbers requiring the service in a given area. Certainly it is advisable to pay bills by bank debit, as reconnection can be extremely slow.

Other regular costs where there is shared ownership include community or service charges. Local rates vary considerably depending upon whether your local town hall is responsible for a city, urbanization or rural area and you should budget for a minimum of 8,000 pesetas upwards. Good insurance cover is essential on your property and this can be obtained from Lloyds of London underwiters for a premium of £2 per £1000 on buildings and £6 per £1000 on contents. Be extremely wary of Spanish policies offering cover of only 5 per cent of damage caused. Many people (including Spanish nationals) who are entitled to free treatment in state hospitals still take out health insurance, as there are long waiting lists for operations. If you are touring Europe or travelling to other countries regularly, health insurance from a British company can be obtained for a premium of around £200 a year, valid in Spain. Maintenance costs for your property should be relatively low, as popular retirement areas are free of dirt in the atmosphere. However, with no cavity walls, repainting with plastic paint at intervals is recommended to prevent damp patches in stormy weather.

Common property   Spain is particularly well organized legally in regard to the administration of property with an element of shared ownership, as there is the *Ley de Propiedad Horizontal* covering connected properties and the *Entidad Urbanística Colaboradora de Conservación y Gestión* for detached villas. A mixed urbanization will decide to be governed by one of these laws. They both provide for the drawing up of local rules covering the convening of meetings, election of officers, preparation of budgets, keeping of accounts, deciding and collecting community charges, besides the use and administration of common property such as stairways, roof spaces, gardens, swimming pools, etc. An Annual General Meeting is held to deal with the above matters, as well as others which arise. Meetings can be conducted in the language which the majority present understand, as long as translation is provided for minorities. Proceedings must be entered in the minute book in Spanish. Contributions are often assessed according to the dimensions of the various properties. The president must be an owner and can be assisted by officials such as administrator, treasurer and secretary, who need not be owners and can be paid. Proxy voting is permitted and you should be on your guard against proxies being collected by an administrator who is the nominee of the developer.

Taxes At the time of writing, various taxation matters are under review in the Spanish parliament. The following is the present position, which comprises interim provisions to accommodate the decision to tax spouses separately. The rules are different for residents and non-residents. Details given are for residents as this book is concerned with retirement abroad and it is therefore assumed that you will spend a total of at least 183 days in Spain (not necessarily continuously) in a calendar year commencing on 1 January, whether or not you have a residence permit. Tax returns must be purchased from a tobacconist and filed (together with payment) in arrears between late May and early June. It is advisable to engage a professional to do this on your behalf, or you could well lose allowances much greater than the small fee charged.

Impuesto sobre la renta de las personas físicas (or *'renta'* for short) is Spanish income tax, which also includes as a separate pool capital gains when realized. No return is required where total income is less than 945,000 pesetas or where investment income is less than 225,000 pesetas per annum. Each year 2 per cent of the official value of any property which you own is added to income. Capital gains are assessed in the year when realized through the sale of assets, after first multiplying the cost of the asset by a coefficient which takes inflation into account, as in the following scale:

Year of Purchase	*Coefficient*
Before 1979	2.559
1979	2.247
1980	1.981
1981	1.762
1982	1.572
1983	1.429
1984	1.311
1985	1.232
1986	1.158
1987	1.114
1988	1.090
1989	1.050
1990	1.000

The resulting adjusted gain is divided by the number of years which have elapsed since the date of purchase. A permanent home which is sold by a taxpayer and produces an adjusted gain of up to 30 million pesetas is subject to exemption providing that the proceeds are used within two years to purchase another principal residence. From 1992 the tax is not payable on a property which you have owned for more than twenty years. The relief is adjusted proportionately if the time limit is exceeded, or if all the proceeds are not used for this purpose. After these adjustments income tax is calculated at the following rates for 1992:

Pesetas from	Pesetas to	Cumulative tax due on amount in above 2nd column	Plus percentage on amount in excess of 1st column
681,300	1,135,500	Nil	25
1,135,500	1,703,250	113,550	26
1,703,250	2,271,000	261,165	27
2,271,000	2,838,750	414,458	28
2,838,750	3,406,500	573,428	30
3,406,500	3,974,250	743,753	32
3,974,250	4,542,000	925,433	34
4,542,000	5,109,750	1,118,468	36
5,109,750	5,677,500	1,322,858	38.5
5,677,500	6,245,250	1,541,441	41
6,245,250	6,813,000	1,774,219	43.5
6,813,000	7,380,750	2,021,190	46
7,380,750	7,948,500	2,282,355	48.5
7,948,500	8,516,250	2,557,714	51
8,516,250	9,084,000	2,847,266	53.5
9,085,000	and over	3,151,013	56

For instance, tax on an assessable income of exactly 1,135,000 pesetas is 113,500 pesetas. On 1,500,000 pesetas it would be 113,500 plus 26 per cent of 364,500 (1,500,000 minus 1,135,500) = 113,500 + 94,770 = 208,270 pesetas.

The resulting tax due is then reduced by various allowances, which are called 'tax credits'. There is an employment income credit of 25,200 pesetas for each wage earner of a family to a maximum of two persons. Additional earners in the same family are entitled to a variable deduction to a maximum of 908,574 pesetas. There is an allowance of 40,000 pesetas for a joint tax declaration by a married couple. A credit of 20,000 pesetas may be taken for each unmarried child under 25 years supported by the taxpayer, 15,000 pesetas for each parent (or other forbears) resident with the taxpayer who is either over seventy years or who earns less than 600,000 pesetas and 50,000 pesetas for each severely handicapped member of the family. If a private residence is purchased then 15 per cent of its cost is deductible. Alternatively, mortgage interest is deductible every year. Life and/or disability insurance attracts a deduction of 10 per cent of the premium if placed with Spanish companies, subject to conditions regarding the term and relationship of beneficiary. Pension plan contributions are allowable to

15 per cent of the amount paid. So is 15 per cent of medical insurance premiums and 15 per cent of substantiated medical expenses. There are two points which expatriates moving to Spain should note. Firstly, they should attempt to complete the purchase of a property between 1 January and 30 June; otherwise the large tax deduction will become due in a year when they are not tax resident in Spain and therefore not due to pay any Spanish income tax. Secondly, although the marginal rate of tax may have appeared to be the same as in Britain at 25 per cent, in fact this is not so, as the tax credits are set against tax due and not against income.

Residents must file a wealth tax (*impuesto extraordinario sobre el patrimonio de las personas físicas*) return if their global assets after deducting charges (such as mortgages) amount to at least 10 million pesetas, property being taken at its official (and not market) value. There is an allowance for residents only of 6 million pesetas for a single person and 9 million pesetas for a married couple. The balance is charged as follows:

Up to 25 million pesetas	0.2%
25 to 50 million pesetas	0.3%
50 to 100 million pesetas	0.45%
100 to 250 million pesetas	0.65%
250 to 500 million pesetas	0.85%
500 to 1000 million pesetas	1.1%
1000 to 1500 million pesetas	1.35%
1500 to 2500 million pesetas	1.7%
Over 2500 million pesetas	2.0%

Inheritance tax (*impuesto sobre sucesiones y donaciones*) is payable between spouses. The method by which it is computed is based upon:

a)   the closeness of the relationship (and sometimes the age) of the beneficiary, on which basic reductions are allowed for three of four classes

b)   the amount inherited

c)   the existing wealth of the beneficiary.

The relationship classes and the relevant allowances are:

Class I:	Descendants and adopted children aged less than 21 years. Allowance – 2,386,000 pesetas, plus 596,000 pesetas for each year under 21.
Class II:	Descendants and adopted children aged over 21 years, spouses, ascendants and adoptants. Allowance – 2,386,000 pesetas.
Class III:	Brothers, sisters, uncles, aunts, nephews, nieces, plus ascendants and descendants by marriage. Allowance – 1,193,000 pesetas.

Class IV: More distant relations and unrelated persons (including common law spouses). Allowance – Nil.

The table of tax rates which is applied after deducting any allowance is as follows:

Value exceeding	Rate %	Excess to	Rate on excess %
0	–	1,193,000	7.65
1,193,000	7.65	1,193,000	8.5
2,386,000	8.08	1,193,000	9.35
3,579,000	8.5	1,193,000	10.2
4,772,000	8.93	1,193,000	11.05
5,965,000	9.35	1,193,000	11.9
7,158,000	9.78	1,193,000	12.75
8,351,000	10.2	1,193,000	13.6
9,544,000	10.63	1,193,000	14.45
10,737,000	11.05	1,193,000	15.3
11,930,000	11.48	5,960,000	16.15
17,890,000	13.03	5,960,000	18.7
23,850,000	14.45	11,925,000	21.25
35,775,000	16.72	23,850,000	25.5
59,625,000	20.23	59,625,000	29.75
119,250,000	24.99	All	34

The final stage of the calculation is to apply the relevant coefficient according to the pre-existing wealth and inheritance class of the heir from the table below:

Existing wealth (million pesetas)	Classes I and II	Class III	Class IV
0 to 60	1	1.5882	2
60 to 300	1.05	1.6676	2.1
300 to 600	1.1	1.7471	2.2
over 600	1.2	1.9059	2.4

At present Spain has double taxation treaties with Austria, Belgium, Brazil, Canada, Czechoslovakia, Denmark, Finland, France, Germany, Italy, Japan, Morocco, Netherlands, Norway, Poland, Portugal, Romania, Sweden, Switzerland and the United Kingdom, although these do not cover inheritance tax. Even where no such convention has been negotiated residents can deduct similar taxes paid abroad from their liability to Spanish tax.

Although not a separate imposition, withholding tax at the rate of 25 per cent is deducted from interest on bank deposit accounts before payment on account of possible income tax due.

Transmission tax (*impuesto sobre transmisiones*) at the current rate of 6 per cent is payable on second-hand dwellings by the purchaser and they are exempted from value added tax.

Strictly speaking, the vendor should pay the *arbitrio sobre increments del valor de los terrenos* (*plus valía* for short) which is a capital gains tax on the increase in value of building land (not structures). It is assessed on a sliding scale from a minimum of 15 per cent where less than five years have elapsed since the previous sale to a maximum of 40 per cent where the period exceeds fifty years.

Value added tax (*impuesto sobre el valor anadido*, or I.V.A. for short) is charged at three differential rates on goods and services which are not exempt. For 1992 the rate is 6 per cent for those regarded as necessities, such as food, medicines, transport and new dwellings; a standard rate of 13 per cent on most items; and 28 per cent on so called luxury items such as all private cars, jewellery, furs, yachts, etc. In 1993 there will only be two rates, 6 per cent and 15 per cent; the loss on motor car revenue being recouped by imposition of a much higher registration tax.

As mentioned earlier, property tax charged by municipal authorities (*contribucíon urbana*) will vary considerably in amount depending upon location and the level of services.

Bank accounts   In regard to the services provided to customers, these are identical whether you bank with a savings bank (*Caja de Ahorros*) or with a commercial bank. Until you apply for a residence permit you are entitled to hold only a non-resident bank account. With resident status you may only have a resident account. Within these classifications current, savings and fixed period deposit accounts are available, with rising rates of interest in that sequence. Spain no longer has exchange control regulations. Residents may have accounts in foreign currencies with Spanish banks. Remember that bank interest due to residents is subject to the deduction before receipt of a 25 per cent withholding tax on account of possible income tax due. When writing cheques it is usual to place the 'numbered' sign (similar to the box used for a game of noughts and crosses) both before and after the figures to prevent alteration. The continental method of separating thousands from smaller units by a full stop and using a comma as a decimal point is followed. When making out a cheque to cash the word *portador* is written as the payee. The maximum amount of cash which a resident may take out of Spain is 1 million pesetas unless form B-3 is completed in the bank.

Residence permits   At present the Spanish authorities show no signs of relaxing the rules regarding residence permits in anticipation of Spain becoming a full member of the European Community on 1 January 1993. In fact, the tendency seems to be the insistence on the transfer of larger monthly sums to Spain than was previously the case. Strictly speaking EC rules will permit community citizens to come to Spain after the above date (a) to seek work (b) to engage in work and (c) to retire in the country after having worked there. There is no automatic right to retire in Spain without previous employment there and it remains to be seen how the authorities will react. Spain needs to attract foreign retired people to help narrow the deficit caused by the adverse trade gap, but it is obviously concerned that those with income of only a small state retirement pension will become a burden. In addition, there is the justifiable suspicion that other EC countries are excessively anxious to unload their responsibilities for the medical and social care of the elderly as the latter become a higher proportion of the population.

That said, the procedure at present for obtaining a residence permit is outlined below. It should be appreciated that local variations will apply in different provinces due to regional autonomy. The first step is to obtain a special visa from a Spanish embassy or consulate in your home country before you leave. Within a maximum of three months from the date of that visa it is necessary to assemble the following documents in Spain:

(a)   your passport with a photocopy of each page up to and including the special visa
(b)   certificate of registration with your local consulate in Spain
(c)   certificate of good conduct from the above consulate
(d)   five passport-type photographs
(e)   the original and a photocopy of your *escritura*, property contract or long-term tenancy agreement.
(f)   evidence of means to support yourself, which is a certificate obtained from your Spanish bank after monthly transfers have been received. The authorities will be looking for a monthly transfer to Spain of at least 114,000 pesetas for a couple or 90,000 pesetas equivalent for a single person.
(g)   confirmation of health cover. For pensioners coming from countries with reciprocal health arrangements this will be confirmation from their health authority, plus registration with the Spanish Health Service. Others need to produce the original and a photocopy of a health insurance policy with a Spanish company or a certificate in Spanish that their foreign policy is valid in Spain.
(h)   fiscal stamps (*papel del estado*) obtained from a state tobacconist to the value of approximately 570 pesetas, depending upon your nationality.

All these papers are taken to the local *Policia Nacional* office and if they are accepted and a receipt given then you are authorized to remain in Spain until the residence permit is issued, which may be up to five months later. An expiry date appears on the *residencia* and it must be renewed in advance.

Local wills   If you die having only a foreign will then the latter will be acted upon in regard to your assets situated in Spain. However, this situation leads to lengthy delays in distributing the estate to the beneficiaries, besides considerable expense in translating and authenticating the foreign will. For these reasons, if no other, it is advisable to have a local will covering your assets situated in Spain and a foreign will for the remainder of your estate. If you wish to make a bequest to a distant relative or to an unrelated person (including common law wife) it is advisable to do so from a foreign will, as you will see from the section on taxation that the donee could lose over 80 per cent of the bequest to Spanish inheritance tax if this provision is made in a Spanish will. It is possible to sign a home made will, although this is not recommended as it could well cause far more expense than it saves, particularly if you inadvertently contravene the Spanish law of obligatory heirs. The recognized procedure to make a local will is to discuss your wishes with a Spanish lawyer or qualified *gestor*, who will then communicate these details to a *notario*. A will is drawn up and you sign this before the latter official. The *notario* sends a report to a central registry in Madrid and keeps the original will. You can retain a photocopy, or an authenticated copy, if you wish.

The amount of detail which can be given on just one country is obviously restricted in an international publication of this kind due to limitations of space. If you are considering retirement in Spain you may wish to read my book entitled *A Villa on the Costa Blanca*, published in London by B.T. Batsford Ltd, ISBN 0-7134-6034-2, price £8.95. This comprehensively covers all aspects of purchasing a property, as well as living and working in Spain in general, plus information specific to the attractive Costa Blanca region. In the case of difficulty the book can be obtained by post from the author's sister Mrs N. Taylor, 13, Dee Avenue, Bellfield, Kilmarnock, Scotland, KA1 3TF, and it will be sent to any country in the world, payment being accepted in any major currency.

UNITED KINGDOM

Climate   Temperate and variable with few settled periods. Temperature rises gradually from 2°C to 6°C in January to 13°C to 22°C in July. Generally colder in Scotland. Rainfall is frequent and unpredictable from an average 37mm in March and April to 64mm in November, with the possibility of heavy thunderstorms in summer. The west is considerably wetter than the east. Damp cold weather is experienced in winter.

Languages   English. Welsh in parts of Wales. Gaelic mostly in the northern regions of Scotland. French is understood by a small minority.

Social customs   Most British people refrain from discussing politics with strangers.

Travel bureaus   There are tourist offices in many large cities throughout the world. The British Council, which is also well represented abroad, can be a good source of information.

Local maps   H.M.S.O., PO Box 276, London SW8 5DT for orders by post, or retail shops in the large provincial cities.

Business hours   Mostly 0900-1300 and 1400-1700 Monday to Friday; with shops, but not offices, open on Saturday.

Inflation   4.3% and falling with mortgage interest included in the calculation.

Local banks   Barclays, Lloyds, Midland, National Westminster and T.S.B. are the main five 'High Street' banks; except in Scotland, where the Royal Bank of Scotland and the Bank of Scotland lead the way.

Precautions & problems   British people, aware of their unsettled weather, are mostly surprised that others would regard their country as a suitable retirement location; although a great many foreigners retire there, attracted by cultural reasons and the variety of entertainment available. The British would also be astounded to learn that their country is a tax haven for foreigners, providing the rules stated below are strictly followed.

House purchase   It is extremely easy to buy a property in Britain at present. In spite of falling markets it would probably be regarded as fairly expensive on a pan-European view. However, prices are likely to be supported after the current recession by steady demand, due to income tax relief being available on interest of mortgages up to £30,000. Prices are highest in London and within a circle around the capital in daily commuting distance. They are lower in northern

England and extremely cheap in northern Scotland if you can bear the climate. There are two main approaches to purchase: either through an estate agent or directly with the seller, contacted from advertisements in regional newspapers or specialist publications such as *Daltons Weekly*. In either case the next step should be to engage a solicitor once you have found a property which suits you. Your solicitor will negotiate with the vendor's legal adviser and they will draw up a contract to the satisfaction of both parties. On completion contracts are exchanged and the title, which has previously been checked, is conveyed to the purchaser. It is usual for your solicitor to arrange insurance cover immediately you are on risk, unless specifically instructed to the contrary. Legally speaking there is nothing to prevent you personally completing the conveyance with the benefit of a 'do-it-yourself' book, although this is not recommended for a foreigner. Most apartments and flats are sold on a long leasehold basis.

Local mortgages   There are a great many building societies with offices in the main commercial areas and the 'High Street' banks also offer loans for property purchase, so you should have no difficulty in obtaining an advance, subject to financial status. If you are going to be liable for British income tax then there are advantages in being able to claim a deduction for mortgage interest payable. It is usual for the lender to conduct a professional survey of the property, for which you will be charged. To rely on this survey to ensure that the property is completely sound may be risky, as the lender is only concerned with value to the extent of the mortgage liability. Suitable insurance cover is likely to be a condition imposed by the lender. The most popular type of mortgage has periodic payments comprising of the interest due plus small repayments of the capital sum.

Planning permission   Planning restrictions are extremely strict and a foreigner would be well advised to delegate such applications to an appropriate professional person, such as an architect. The latter profession has an extremely high standard of conduct as well as expertise and it is very unlikely that you would be disappointed if you left all matters such as design, materials, selection of quantity surveyor and builder to the architect, providing that you supply full details of your requirements and budget, besides approving the plans after careful study. The architect will oversee the construction at all stages and provide certificates of satisfactory work at intervals, against which instalment payments are made. If this extends over a fair period and your income does not arise in sterling, then remember to take independent financial advice on how best to protect yourself from adverse currency fluctuations.

Utilities, costs & maintenance   Water is invariably drinkable and a mains supply is available in practically every area. There may be temporary restrictions on the use of hosepipes in certain localities during drought conditions. In 1990 water costs increased on average in Britain by 19 per cent due to the combination of privatisation of utilities, reduction in subsidies and pressure from the European Community to improve quality. Charges vary due to independent pricing by regional companies, but can be taken to amount to around £0.37 per cubic metre, which is a little less than the average for Western European countries.

Electricity Boards for the various regions were previously part of a nationalized monopoly, but these have recently been privatised. A supply is available at 240 volts virtually everywhere in Britain. The use of electricity for space heating can prove to be extremely expensive in winter and alternatives are to be recommended, although night storage heaters can be operated at a much lower off-peak rate.

Mains gas is available in a great many urban areas and its cost is less than electricity for all purposes. Butane gas can be obtained for around £12 per cylinder and this can provide portable heating in the location desired.

Quite a few properties have oil-fired central heating and the cost of heating oil will obviously vary with the current market price of a barrel of oil.

Considerably more use of coal is made for domestic purposes in Britain than most countries elsewhere, although many urban areas have been declared 'smoke-free' zones. However, various types of smokeless coal are available.

Mains drainage is available virtually everywhere, except in extremely remote areas.

Telephone installation is completed in almost all locations with the minimum of delay.

Other costs include the community charge (or 'poll tax') which is imposed by all local authorities to cover their costs. Naturally this varies enormously according to the services provided and you should budget in the region of £160 to £360 per person a year, until it is replaced by a different charge. Obviously your property and its contents should be insured and the free services of an insurance broker to obtain the best rates can be utilized, if cover has not already been arranged by your solicitor on purchase of the property. As modern building is subject to strict supervision during construction it is not likely that maintenance costs will be high; although expenditure on heat insulation may be necessary, which is likely to be economic.

Common property   Britain differs from continental Europe in that apartments and flats are mostly sold on a long leasehold and seldom freehold. When such properties are rented it is usual for the tenancy agreement to set out in detail the responsibilities of the tenants and to state exactly what common services the landlord will provide.

Taxes The following are details of the British taxation system as set out in the 1992/93 fiscal year budget proposals. Each person can have an annual income of £3,445 before coming into the taxable range. The married couples' additional allowance is £1,720. There are slightly larger personal and married couples' allowances for the 65 to 74 years age group of £4,200 and £2,465 respectively and even greater ones for the over 75 years olds of £4,370 and £2,515. The basic rate of income tax remains at 25 per cent. However, a new lower band will be introduced for the first £2,000 of income at 20 per cent and the basic rate levied on the next £21,700 of taxable income; above which figures the higher rate of 40 per cent applies.

Mortgage interest relief on property loans of up to £30,000 can now be claimed at the standard rate of 25 per cent.

In the case of Capital Gains Tax the annual exemption limit is £5,800 per person. It is charged as if it represents an addition to income, after indexation strips out the effects of inflation. This tax is not levied upon the sale of a property which is deemed to be your principal private residence.

Inheritance Tax is not charged on assets passing between spouses, otherwise the first £150,000 is free of this tax and the excess is charged at 40 per cent. Gifts made more than seven years before death are exempted and there is a sliding scale of reduced charges for gifts during the period of three to seven years before death.

Value Added Tax was raised on 1 April 1991 from 15 to 17.5 per cent. Food and some other categories of goods and services are either exempt from VAT or zero rated.

Previously householders paid rates to the local authority, although this was replaced in 1990 by a Community Charge (poll tax) per head fixed independently by each authority. The 1991 budget reduced the charge by £140 per person. The abolition of the unpopular Community Charge has since been announced. This is to be replaced in 1993 by a Council Tax based upon property values in eight tiers, with a 25 per cent reduction for single occupants and people on a low income. Meanwhile it is advisable to budget upon an annual Community Charge of up to £360 per person, depending upon area of residence.

An outline of the British fiscal system was given in Chapter 29. Foreigners coming to live in the UK should take careful note of the very favourable tax-free environment mentioned in that chapter for foreign residents who retain their original domicile; which will be the case in the vast majority of instances, because it is extremely difficult to change your domicile under the fiscal rules. Be extremely careful to set up three separate and quite distinct bank accounts for (a) income (b) capital gains and (c) pure capital, so that you can live solely on the latter to escape UK taxation on remittances from another country.

Bank accounts Although there are no restrictions on foreigners opening bank accounts in the UK, you will probably be asked to supply a bank reference and a personal reference. There are three main types of accounts; (a) current (called a checking account by Americans), which bears no interest (b) deposit, with which no cheque book is supplied and interest is typically around 6 per cent below the official bank rate and (c) high interest cheque account, with interest of perhaps only 1½ per cent below the bank rate. It is now possible to arrange gross payment of interest upon signature of a declaration of non-liability to UK income tax. As this may well pose complications for resident foreigners they are probably best advised to open accounts with branches located in the Channel Islands or the Isle of Man, where this difficulty does not arise. Remember to have all interest credited to an income account and not to one consisting solely of capital gains or capital, otherwise their purity will become impaired.

Residence permits The subject of immigration to the UK for non-EC citizens has become quite complicated and it is not possible to summarise it in a book such as this one. If you are contemplating coming to live in Britain then you are advised to contact your nearest British Embassy or Consulate for details of the requirements in your individual circumstances. Residence in the Channel Islands is almost impossible, unless you are extremely wealthy.

Local wills Making a will in the UK can be a very informal matter and will forms can be purchased at many stationers. However, you are strongly cautioned against this likely false economy. It is advisable to consult a solicitor (preferably one with an international clientele), so that the ramifications of residence in one country and domicile in another can be thoroughly explored in relation to the fiscal considerations of this complicated situation.

Further Reading

Also published by Robert Hale

Living in France Philip Holland
Living in Italy Yve Menzies
Living in Spain John Reay-Smith
Living in Portugal Susan Thackeray

Index